Fitnotism

Allison Staley C.Ht.

Ryan Staley C.Ht.

ISBN:0692587403
ISBN-13:9780692587409

DEDICATION

To anyone who knows what they should be doing but struggles with
actually doing it

CONTENTS

ACKNOWLEDGMENTS

We want to thank the hundreds of clients who have trusted us to help them lose weight. Your hard work helped inspire this book. We also want to thank Sharon C. Warren for her copy editing services.

INTRODUCTION

It's hard to come back from weight loss failure. There's that gnawing feeling that once you've failed, success somehow is out of reach for you; that your failure to lose weight or keep the pounds off, means that you're doomed to fail again and again. Don't believe it, though! You can learn from your mistakes and turn past dieting failures into one gigantic mega success. You can achieve a healthy slim body and be in control of your eating.

Everyone fails at one time or another, in fact, nothing of worth has ever come without a price. Success takes work and resiliency. Standing among the ruins of past efforts, feeling a bit beaten, you can realize that here in the wreckage you are actually stronger. You have gained valuable experience from that failure. You are now stronger, wiser and far more experienced than you were when you failed. Failure is okay, it means you were trying something. Try often enough, one of those paths will eventually lead to success. Especially if you are able to notice what didn't work about what you attempted the first time...and then you try something different.

Weight loss is the perfect example of these truths. It can be hard to stick to a diet and, once a diet ends, it is all too easy to go back to your old way of eating; the old way that caused you to be heavier than you ever expected in the first place. Pounds creep on and then you fight to battle them off... over and over. Still, finding yourself heavier than you want to be after all that effort and all those diets can be not only frustrating but depressing, too. It can lead to people completely giving up on their dreams of ever maintaining a healthy lifestyle.

But, what if there was another way? What if there were new information and research on the subject of dieting and weight loss?

What if that information could prove that you had simply been attempting the wrong things, that you had been putting your focus on the wrong things? What if, with the right techniques, focus and actions you could accomplish all your goals and more? Achieving those goals is just about digging deeper than the basic conventional wisdom and finding the right steps to lead you to ultimate and ongoing success. That's what this book is about!

My goal is to encourage you to the point that you'll be willing to try again to lose weight and keep it off. I want to let you know that you can accomplish your goals and that this time will be different, because you are going to have the right information and tools to make it different. This is going to be like no diet you've ever been on because there is NO diet. It's a series of simple lifestyle modifications that will help you start to eat less and have more control over your cravings. These steps will help make your weight loss almost automatic and help you save your willpower for only those most tempting of occasions and holidays.

The secret is this one simple truth. Research has proven that losing weight and keeping it off is really all about creating the right environment, habits and mindset. The rest will take care of itself.

In fact, scientists studying weight loss have found that making small modifications to your surroundings and having the right habits actually helps people lose more weight and keep it off better than trying to stick to any certain diet. In fact, simply being aware of how your mind works as it relates to food choices and then using that information to your advantage has been proven to help you consistently lose weight.

HOW THIS BOOK WAS CREATED

My husband and I are both certified personal trainers with

years of experience in the health, fitness and weight loss industry. We own three gyms and have used exercise to help hundreds of people reshape their bodies, but we ran into one frustrating truth. Over and over again, we found we could tell someone exactly what they needed to do to get healthy, workout and have a great diet plan, but they just couldn't do it. For whatever reason, they'd stop coming into the gym, they'd go off their diets and they'd start to give up on maintaining a healthy lifestyle.

We watched as client after client struggled to lose weight, and eventually gained it back again. We have been frustrated seeing that about 15 percent of the people who come in and buy a gym membership, never come in and use it. This frustration has led us to finally admit to ourselves that something about the "traditional" way of doing things just isn't working.

We wanted our clients to succeed long term. We wanted them to get in shape with our training and then stay in shape. We wanted them to eat healthy for more than just a couple of weeks. We started to realize even though we were giving out expert advice, providing personalized dietitian design meal plans and standing over people making them workout, something was missing. We had to admit to ourselves that part of weight loss and exercise success really is mental and to get people the long term results we wanted to give them, we would have to address that piece of the weight loss equation. We wanted to find a way to "fix" our clients thinking and make them think differently.

My husband and I did our research and found the only nationally accredited school for hypnotherapy in the country, The Hypnosis Motivation Institute. We took several introductory classes, passed a test and then applied to be accepted into the full program. Once we got in, we completed hundreds of hours of course work and were eventually awarded the title of master hypnotists. We joined the American Hypnosis Association as professional hypnotherapists and started using our background and training to help people lose weight in a whole new way.

We have been very successful in helping hundreds of clients, many of whom have lost 50 to 60 pounds or more. Best of all, these clients are keeping the weight off better than the majority of our past personal training clients and have made lifelong improvements to their health. We opened a clinic for weight loss hypnosis called Fitnotism and now combine our personal training with hypnosis for incredible results!

Our clients have had so much success we wanted to make our best tips, secrets and knowledge available to everyone. Our background is very unique and that has enabled us to see what really works with our clients and gym members. Now we are passing on that knowledge to you.

PROOF HYPNOSIS IS EFFECTIVE FOR WEIGHT LOSS

You can trust that this will work for you if you are at all suggestible to hypnosis. Why? Because hypnosis for weight loss has been widely studied and documented. In fact, study after study has proven hypnosis can help dieters lose more weight and keep it off longer when compared to other dieters who were not hypnotized.

Many of these studies have been conducted by clinical psychologists and are on record with the US National Library of Medicine - National Institutes of Health. If you want to look them up you can find the information online at PubMed.gov. One of the first major studies on the effectiveness of hypnosis was published in the Journal of Clinical Psychology in 1985 by Bolocofsky, Spinler, and Coulthard-Morris. It studied the effect of adding hypnosis to a behavioral weight loss program. The researchers had 109 subjects who were given professional help to change their eating behavior. Some of these people also underwent hypnosis, others did not. The diets were well designed and successful. Both groups lost significant amounts of weight but, at the 8 month and 2 year follow-up points, those who also got the hypnosis showed significant additional weight loss, while the other group did not. Also, the people who underwent the added hypnosis achieved and then maintained their weight loss goals. Simply put, both groups lost some weight when put on a good, sensible diet but those using hypnosis continued losing weight after the structured diet ended and then continued to keep it off.

Why? Because, unlike those who were only on a diet, their thinking had actually changed.

Another study on the effectiveness of hypnosis for long term weight loss appeared in the Journal of Consulting and Clinical Psychology in 1995 by Kirsch, Montgomery, and Sapirstein. This was an analysis of 18 different studies where cognitive-behavioral therapy was compared to that same therapy when it was supplemented by hypnosis. The results showed that adding hypnosis substantially improved treatment outcomes. In fact, the average client who got cognitive-behavioral hypnotherapy showed greater improvement than at least 70% of clients who received the non-hypnotic cognitive-behavioral therapy treatment. They found that these effects were particularly pronounced for treatments of obesity, especially when it came to sustained long-term weight loss.

In 1996, another study on the effectiveness of hypnosis appeared in Psychological Reports by Johnson and Karkut. It focused specifically on women's weight loss. In this study, the researchers followed a total of 172 overweight adult women. They treated 86 of them with hypnosis only and 86 of them with hypnosis and aversion therapy, such as electric shock and disgusting tastes and smells. They found that both programs achieved significant weight loss. The addition of aversion therapy did not provide any significant improvement in the client outcomes.

In 2001, Scientific American announced that, because of the evidence found in these earlier studies and others like them, a task force from the American Psychological Association had officially validated hypnosis as an adjunct treatment for obesity. That means that, in the serious cases reviewed in these studies, expert diet and exercise advice was crucial; but, when it was supplemented with behavioral hypnotherapy the results were significantly greater and more long lasting. These studies make it clear that to achieve maximum long-term weight loss it is important to use both a diet and exercise program combined with a behavioral hypnotherapy program. In short, the goal is to change people's behaviors by changing the way they think about food and exercise both on a conscious and subconscious level.

GETTING MAXIMUM RESULTS

The results you notice after implementing mental, environmental and hypnotic techniques for weight loss start with a whisper. It's a slight feeling of having more control and a little extra motivation. Soon the real changes begin. You look at a slice of pizza, but somewhere in your mind you just don't feel the need to have three pieces anymore. It's not that the pizza doesn't look appetizing; it's just somehow a little less appealing. Now, one small slice and a salad somehow sound better. Your mind seems to believe that your stomach wouldn't feel as heavy and as greasy that way-- three pieces just seems like too much.

Hypnosis has a beneficial effect when it comes to exercise, too. First you may notice the concept of exercising actually doesn't sound that bad. Where you may have actively not wanted to work-out in the past, now you feel a bit more open to it. Slowly your mind begins working on the issue, starting to come up with options for exercise that could work with your lifestyle and schedule. Eventually, you decide it just feels natural to give your chosen workout a try. You notice it feels better than you had thought it would and better than you had perhaps experienced in the past. You may falter a bit starting out, doing a few days here and a few days there. Over time, as the repetition continues, you begin to realize how much better both your body and mind feel when you are being active and you find yourself working out more, become the kind of person who is moving more every day.

Amazingly, you will find that same thing happening with French fries, desserts, and sweet drinks. It's not that they aren't appealing anymore. They still sound good. The difference is that you really can stop after having just a little bit of them. The change is that you don't feel compelled to polish off the entire serving and crave even more. You notice at a dinner party that you feel more in control at the buffet table. It's not that the rich, heavy, sweet, creamy food isn't there, or that it doesn't look good to you. It's that you just don't feel like you HAVE to have it anymore. You might have a spoonful or two of it, but that is enough to satisfy you. You don't find yourself going into an eating frenzy and overeating just because it's there. You no longer feel the urge to eat until you are stuffed. You are in control now and food just doesn't look THAT good. And that's when you realize the hypnosis is starting to work.

Hypnosis isn't magic that can make all sweets suddenly seem disgusting forever. No, it's just a subtle change in your thinking that allows the pounds to slowly disappear over time. What accomplishes these small shifts in thinking is repetitively listening to the weight loss hypnosis commands while at the hypnotherapist office and on a CD before you go to bed at night, since that is when the mind is most open to self-hypnosis. You could say hypnotherapy programs are one of those things in life where, "It only works if you work it." The more you listen to your personalized recordings and allow yourself to go deeply into a hypnotic state, the more subtle things you'll begin to notice changing in your life.

For example, one client's goal was to drink more water. She knew water is one of life's building blocks and that it would make her skin look better and help her keep from snacking. During professional hypnosis sessions, she was told repeatedly that she would drink more water. "Water will be there to help you lose the weight," she was told. At first she didn't believe it was working. She still wasn't a fan of plain water. She didn't have any desire to drink a big tall glass of ice water. She was frustrated until she stopped for a moment and thought. She realized she was drinking more warm tea than ever before. She was drinking it at night to relax. Then during the day, she always seemed to need a cup of warm tea in her hand. It was so natural she hadn't even noticed the change until she started thinking about how those suggestions to drink more water had failed. At that moment she realized they hadn't failed at all. She was getting 8 to 10 glasses of water a day, her skin was better and she was snacking less. Her subconscious mind, as it's prone to do, took those suggestions to drink more water and acted upon them, in a way consistent with her subconscious programming. This client believed she didn't like cold plain ice water much, but she was fine with warm tea. It was just a subtle change but the hypnotic suggestions enabled her shift her behavior to achieve her goal.

If these subtle changes are held back, or if these habits are abandoned right after they appear, all the good done by hypnosis can be undone. For example, if the client mentioned above had decided that the extra tea was making her have to run to the bathroom too often and if she made a conscious effort to stop drinking it, soon that new fledgling tea habit would disappear. However, if she encouraged it and gave in to that healthy urge every time she felt it, the habit would become more and more ingrained in her lifestyle.

In short, the results gained from the use of mental, environmental and hypnotic techniques are small, subtle and cumulative. Over time and with encouragement, they can add up to a massive shift in lifestyle. Even scientific studies have shown that dieters using weight loss hypnosis have been able to keep the weight off better than dieters just using diet alone because of these changes in thinking. One session, plus at home listening to personalized CD's, typically will aid in relaxation and general weight loss motivation. It can also potentially create a few subtle shifts in thinking that may be noticeable. As more sessions are added, those subtle shifts in thinking begin to add up, becoming even more apparent and becoming even more deeply ingrained. Results from hypnotherapy are often felt throughout a lifetime, becoming a natural part of client's lives.

SKINNY SECRET 1: GOOD HABITS CONSERVE YOUR WILLPOWER

There are a million diets out there and if one doesn't work out, there is always another one around the corner. From pills to powders to Garcinia Cambogia and shots, there's always something new to try. The trap is that people seem to think the solution to their big problem with weight needs to be something expensive, important and complicated, like a "secret" they just need to uncover. Here's the secret… all diets work to some extent. Whether it's Gluten Free, Sugar-Free, Fat-Free, or Carb Free, it doesn't matter which you choose, you'll lose weight as long as you have the willpower to stick with it.

For too many people, though, willpower is something mysterious. It is a force of self-control that sometimes is with them going strong and at other times seems to desert them completely. It is fickle, making them think they are in control and easily able to lose weight and then it seems to just evaporate.

Now it's time for you to solve that mystery once and for all. Willpower has actually been studied numerous times over the years by researchers looking at who has it, when they use it and how often it is applied. What they've found is that while it is true that some people do tend to be better a delaying gratification than others, in general, willpower is like a resource in our bodies. We seem to only have so much of it and once it gets used up, we tend to get a lot worse at stopping our impulse for instant gratifications.

Research has also found that people, who want to lose weight but don't have a daily plan of exactly what meals they're going to eat tend to lose less weight and be less successful that people who do have an eating plan.

If you take these two findings and look at them together,

you'll begin to see what is actually causing people to fail in their weight loss attempts. When someone doesn't have a plan about what they are going to eat, they have to consider all their options and then chose the healthiest one. Making that "right" choice takes willpower. In fact, they end up have to exercise that will power over and over again every time they make any food choice. So, when they are faced with an unexpected temptation, like someone bringing donuts to the office, they will be far more likely to give into that temptation. They have simply run out of willpower.

It has been proven that someone who is following a plan will be less likely to eat the donuts at the office. In fact, it doesn't even matter too much what type of plan it is. It could be they are following a specific diet or maybe they just have a meal plan they came up with on their own. It doesn't matter. They are going through their day knowing what they will eat and how much they will eat. They haven't had to use their willpower to make tons of meal decisions. That's why, when the donuts get to the office, they still have enough willpower to not have one.

The studies have gone even further, showing that people who eat the same meals over and over tend to lose weight more effectively than those who are constantly changing it up. Variety might be the spice of life but, unfortunately, it can lead to extra weight gain.

You can make these findings work for you by coming up with your own meal plan. Maybe it's that you have scrambled eggs for breakfast, a salad or soup for lunch and then chili, grilled chicken kabobs or shrimp for dinner. You can test this yourself. Plan out your meals and your snacks and eat mostly the same few meals over and over; you will find you lose more weight! My point is that it doesn't matter what the meals are, as long as they're light enough to help you lose weight. It's the repetition and the lack of thought you have to put into it that causes you to have willpower when you really need it. That extra willpower causes extra weight loss.

There is another truth at play when it comes to deciding to follow some sort of eating plan. It's a simple mental technique called "pattern disrupt." Pattern disrupt works for any new diet that's different from how you've eaten in the past because it's disrupting your normal pattern of eating. It causes you to watch what you eat and so, of course, at least a few pounds will drop off regardless of what plan you're following. In conclusion, it's not about finding that one perfect diet.

After two decades of experience in the fitness industry and thousands of clients, my husband and I have seen that a few diets are slightly more effective than others. We've found that clients who lost the most weight, the quickest, were doing HCG Drops or The Atkins Diet. Neither is particularly healthy and neither is a great long term solution. Still, if we had to pick the top two diets that work quickly, those would be them. We can't recommend the HCG drops though because they are a hormone drop and the long-term effects of that are questionable. We have seen the drops successfully kill the appetites of numerous people, allowing them to follow the HCG 500 calorie a day diet.

We don't recommend that you follow that 500 calorie a day diet. Your body needs at least 1,000 calories a day to function. If it doesn't get that it burns not only your fat for energy but also your muscles. YOUR MUSCLES ARE YOUR METABOLISM. IF YOU BURN THEM, YOUR METABOLISM IS RUINED! You burn your muscles, you will regain all the weight you've lost, plus lots of extra weight. The Atkins Diet does work to lose weight. It involves eliminating almost all carbohydrates from your diet. On Atkins, you can kiss fruit, juice, bread and pasta good-bye. It does, however, allow you to have tons of bacon, cream and butter. Obviously this is hard on the system and, long term, probably isn't great for your heart health. Please, whatever diet or eating style you choose, just eat healthily and focus on avoiding processed foods.

SKINNY SECRET 2: SEE RED TO EAT LESS

Did you know that researchers believe that making small subliminal changes in your daily lifestyle is actually more effective at causing long-term weight loss than any diet that requires willpower?

In fact, what if I told you about one psychological experiment that, if you take advantage of its findings, could make you 10 to 20 pounds thinner in just one year? It's true! Researchers have looked at every detail of the way you eat and found there is a magic recipe to eating less. Crazy right? Just make your table, fork and plates look the right way and you'll instantly eat less.

Here is research behind the magical Delboeuf illusion, that one experiment than can help you drop major weight effortlessly. Basically, it shows that your eyes really do play tricks on you. All one Belgian researcher, named Joseph Delboeuf, did was create two black dots that were the same size and then he drew a different sized circle around each of them. One circle was smaller than the other. Interestingly people looking at his drawing thought the dots were a different size. In fact, people saw the dot that had the larger circle around it as being smaller.

Simply put, this translates to weight loss because your plate acts just like Delboeuf's ring and your food acts just like his dot. If you put your food on a larger plate your mind will automatically see the amount of food on it as being smaller. If you put your food on a smaller plate, your mind will automatically see the amount of food on it as being larger.

The red plate idea comes from Swiss researchers. They gave people either red, white or blue plates and cups with either a red or blue sticker. Those who had the red plates and cups ended up eating and drinking significantly less than those who used the blue or the white. The researchers interpreted their results as meaning that red means stop subconsciously to people, causing them to stop eating.

Two researchers, Dr. Brian Wansink and Dr. Koert van Ittersum, at Cornell University took the Swiss researcher's work one step further. They played a trick on people at a buffet giving some of them a red plate and others a white plate at an all you can eat pasta bar. On the buffet, there was either Alfredo sauce pasta or Marinara sauce pasta. They then secretly weighed everyone's plate with hidden scales. The folks who had the red plates and chose the Marinara pasta and the folks who had the white plates and chose the Alfredo pasta piled on way more food. Those who picked the pasta in the color that contrasted with the color of their plate piled on a lot less, 22 percent less to be exact. Thus the two researchers proved, if you're eating Alfredo, don't put it on a white plate, and if you are eating something red, that is the one time you wouldn't want to use a red plate. The color of your plate should always be different than the color of the food you are eating.

These same researchers also found that if your plate is the same color as your tablecloth, you'll also serve yourself a lot less. Those who had a red plate on a red table cloth or a white plate on a white tablecloth tended to pile on 10 percent less. So put simply, their eating research proves you'll eat less if you eat while seeing a bunch of red... except in cases where the food you are eating also happens to be red.

SUPER SIZE YOUR FORK

Here is one more sneaky trick to get your mind to do the work for you when losing weight. You just need to super size your fork. This information comes from Italian researchers who studied two groups of people eating the same meal.

They gave one group big forks and the other group small forks. The group with the smaller forks ate significantly more. When asked why they thought this happened, people reported feeling like they weren't getting their hunger satisfied with the small forks.

Apparently small forks are just less satisfying than big forks. So if you want your hunger satisfied more quickly, causing you to eat less, use a smaller fork.

SKINNY DINNER COMPANIONS CAN MAKE YOU FAT

You'll want watch out for those pesky skinny dinner companions. Did you know that if you are eating with someone who is skinny but is really chowing down on a ton of food, it will make you far more likely to overeat? A skinny person packing away fork full after fork full sends the unconscious message that you too can eat a lot without the calories really counting. Research has shown you will automatically eat more if you're eating with this type of companion.

In fact, skinny people with a big appetite are the most dangerous dinner accessory if you're trying to drop a few pounds. The best dinner companion is actually a normal to a heavy set man with a fairly small appetite. Research has shown that, particularly if you're a woman, you'll naturally eat less around men. It's strange but true, and it happens automatically.

SKINNY SECRET 3: COPY GOOGLE'S KITCHEN DESIGN

Everyone already knows that Google is awesome. It is a great search engine, a cool tech company and a major employer. Who knew it can also help keep us thin? They've proven that certain mental tricks when it comes to kitchen layout can work to help people cut major calories without even having to think about it. Unlike other older, less progressive companies, instead of telling their workers to eat healthier and handing out some generic guide about what healthy foods are, like broccoli and chicken breast, Google just hid the junk food. No joke! They put the salad and fruit front and center at their cafeteria and moved the junk food off onto a bottom shelf in an opaque box...and boom! People instantly started eating better.

In fact, Google actually tracked the change and found that their workers ate nearly 10 percent less candy over the course of a week with just that one simple change. It's amazing how much we humans just go with what's easiest to grab without even thinking about it. As you have probably noticed when wondering if you remembered to put the garage door down or turn off the stove, we spend a lot of our lives on autopilot. That is also true of how we eat. We all too often eat and drink on autopilot. We often don't even think about what we're putting in our mouths, because our minds are busy concentrating on our relationships, our goals or even just our shopping list. Google took advantage of this natural phenomenon. Then, Google got even bigger results just by making the bottled water super accessible, putting it on a front and center shelf and bumping the sodas down to a lowly bottom shelf. Most of the time people just grabbed the first thing they saw.

Google tracked the results and found they'd bumped up their employees bottled water consumption by an astonishing 47 percent while reducing the amount of soda the employees drank. Way to go Google! Obviously, you can get these same great results in your own home by doing exactly the same thing. Put a big bowl of fruit on your kitchen counter. Make sure to have some washed, cut up veggies front and center in the fridge and a big jug of water, tea or bottled water on the counter top. You'll want to hide the junk food from yourself in a non-see-through container on the bottom shelf of your pantry and put the soda way in the back of the fridge. That's all the effort it takes and research has proven… YOU WILL EAT FEWER CALORIES.

Bottom line, all it takes to eat better is putting the foods you wish you'd eat in easy reach and making those naughty foods you'd want to stay away from harder to get to.

GOOGLE YOUR CLOSET

You can also use your closet to help you drop weight without really thinking about it. Find your "skinny clothes" those clothes that look best when you're at your lightest weight and put them front and center. You can even hang them on the front of your closet door. Simply seeing them over and over again is a great way to give your subconscious and your motivation a little boost.

SKINNY CLOTHES HYPNOSIS

Imagine your skinny clothes, hanging there in the back of your closet. Those clothes, pants, skirt, bathing suit, that special wardrobe item that's so you. It would look so good, be so gorgeous on you, if only you could fit into it. How long has it been hanging there waiting for you, months, years? How long has it been since you felt really good, good enough to put it on, good enough to plan to wear it out? It's time to get back to that place, that moment. It's time to give yourself that gift. Visualize yourself taking those skinny clothes out of the closet and hanging them on your bathroom door. You can see them every time you walk into the bathroom, every time you get out of the shower, every time you go to do your hair or brush your teeth. Every time you see them, those skinny clothes, you say to yourself, "That's where I'm going, that's where I'm going." You find yourself starting to point at them. "That's where I'm going. That's where I'm going." Every time you are about to get the cookies, every time you consider running out for a hamburger, every time you're about to shove a handful of chips into your mouth, you go back and look at that door. You see your skinny clothes. You point. You repeat, "That's where I'm going." "That's where I'm going." And, you believe that's where you're going; you know you will fit into them. And you know when you do, you are going to look amazing. You are going to feel proud, confident and ready to take on the world. You look at those clothes saying, "That's where I'm going. That's where I'm going." And, you believe it. You know that's the truth. That's where you are going. Every day, that's where you are going.

SKINNY SECRET 4: GIVE YOURSELF A MENTAL EDGE

What if I told you there is a test that takes less than 10 minutes, doesn't hurt and can cause you to lose weight and keep it off. According to research done benefiting the U.S. Military, there is such a test and it's called an RMR, or a resting metabolic rate test. You actually burn the majority of your daily calories, 60-75 percent, without even thinking about it. It's burned by your muscles and used to keep you living and breathing. Everyone's body is different and requires a different number of calories to maintain its simple daily functions. That number of calories is known as your metabolic fingerprint. It is based on science known as your resting metabolic rate. Research shows just knowing your resting metabolic rate can help you better understand your body's true caloric needs and cause you to naturally eat less.

Here's how it works. It takes a certain amount of oxygen in order to burn one calorie. If you were to measure exactly how much oxygen your body is using over a 24 hour period, you would find out how many calories it burned. That then would be your magic number, the number of calories you could eat while laying in bed doing absolutely nothing and not gain a single pound. While there are mathematical equations you can use to guess your metabolic fingerprint, they tend to be rather inaccurate. They are based on a bell curve and many people don't fall exactly where they are theoretically supposed to. Therefore, going to a doctor's office, gym or another provider and getting an accurate number is worth the money. It usually costs only about $100.

The number is very powerful because once you know it, suddenly you are in control. You know what you need to survive and can factor in your movement and exercise. If you eat less than what you are burning, your RMR, you will lose weight, if you eat more, you will gain weight. You'll know if you really do have a slow metabolism or if you actually have a pretty fast one. This can be life changing. One woman in her early 30's, who is roughly 5'9", kept gaining weight. She was eating healthy things like oatmeal with raisins and walnuts for breakfast. Her dinners were made up of chicken, whole grain pasta and sweet potatoes. The problem was her metabolic fingerprint showed she had a slow metabolism and only burned 1200 calories a day.

Even with moderate movement added in, if she didn't exercise, she needed to eat less than 1400 calories a day just to avoid gaining any weight. Though she had been eating healthy, her diet was made up of very calorie dense foods like bread, pasta, potatoes and dried fruit. Since she was relatively young and tall, she had been drastically over-estimating the amount of healthy food and fuel her body needed, causing her to gain weight. Once we knew her RMR, we switched her to foods that were less calorie dense.

On the other end of the spectrum we found a 66-year-old woman, who was only 5 feet tall had a metabolic fingerprint of 1510 calories a day. She had been unable to stick to the very low-calorie diets she had been put on in the past and had dropped out of very low-calorie prepackaged meal programs. She swung back and forth between restrictive dieting and then out of control eating. Her metabolic fingerprint revealed why she was failing on the diets and then finding it almost impossible to resist binge-eating. She required 1510 calories a day to run her body, so when she was put on very calorie restrictive diets her body would go into starvation mode, she would start to feel fuzzy headed and sluggish until she ultimately gave up and gave her body the calories it needed to survive. The binges were brought on by a real physical need for more food, but after binge-eating she would feel like a failure and overdo it. By finding out her metabolic fingerprint, she then understood that she simply needed a moderate calorie meal plan to avoid her pattern of dieting, failing and binge-eating.

Even if you don't have access to an RMR test, I can give you a good idea of what your RMR would likely be. I have done hundreds and hundreds of RMR tests for our gym and Fitnotism clients and can often predict the results fairly closely just by talking to someone. Your RMR is likely 1000 or below if you have an untreated thyroid problem, have been on bed rest for an extended period of time (causing muscle deterioration) or if you have been eating less than 1000 calories for an extended period of time. You need to eat at least 1000 calories a day or your body starts burning your muscle and your fat. Burning your muscle tanks your metabolism.

Your RMR is likely around 1200 if you tend to carry very little muscle mass, struggle with losing weight when dieting and you are female. Most women we see with this type of RMR tend to be small to medium boned, average to plump body types and are 45 or older. Some women who are younger but were never athletic and even struggled with their weight as children tend to be about this RMR.

Your RMR is likely 1400 if you are an average woman in your 20's, 30's or 40's. If you were thinner as a child, lose weight fairly easily when dieting or tend to carry more muscle mass than the average women, you may even be around 1400 for your RMR in your 50's or 60's. Women who have 50 pounds or more to lose often have an RMR of at least 1400.

If you are a woman who has well over 50 pounds to lose, always lost weight easily or was very athletic not too long ago, your RMR may be 1600 calories a day. Men who carry very little muscle mass or are older and mostly inactive but still fairly average sized may have an RMR of 1600 calories.

If you are a man and are fairly active, carry a decent amount of muscle, were active when you were younger or have about 20 pounds or more to lose, you may have an RMR of 1800 calories. If you are a large man, have a stocky muscular body, were active when you were young and have 50 pounds or more to lose you may even have an RMR somewhere just above 2000 calories a day.

Please note, eating the same amount of calories your body burns at rest will not cause you to lose much weight if you lead a mostly inactive lifestyle. You have to create a calorie deficit to lose weight. That means if you are being mostly inactive, you need to eat about 200 calories less than your RMR to lose weight at any kind of a decent pace.

Never eat below 1000 calories though because doing so will tank your metabolism. If you have an RMR around 1000 calories you will have to burn an extra 200 calories with moderate exercise while eating 1000 calories a day to lose weight. If you are in this situation, you may have a thyroid condition and may want to consult your physician or you may need to build more muscle.

RMR SELF HYPNOSIS

Your mind has been lying to you. Your mind has been fooling you. Telling you that you need heavy foods. Telling you that you need bigger meals or that you should eat very often. It tells you that you need to eat enough to make sure you get all the nutrients you need. That you need substantial food so you don't get hungry or waste away.

These messages are all lies. You now realize your body has a smaller metabolism. It only requires a small amount of calories.

(Repeat your RMR Magic Number)

As you have gotten older your metabolism has slowed. Your metabolism is now slower but steady. It handles lighter foods best. You realize you only need a small amount of calories each day.

(Repeat your RMR Magic Number)

Large amounts of your favorite heavy foods like .... donuts, pizza, pasta, cookies, ice cream, French fries, chips or chocolate are too heavy. These things are too calories dense for your body to burn efficiently. Eating these foods puts on fat. Your metabolism easily and effectively burns fresh fruits and vegetables, lean meats, lean dairy and only small amounts of whole grains. When you eat rich heavy foods, some of those calories stay with you.

Those foods are so calorie dense. Your body can only burn off some of their calories. The rest stays with you as fat. Some people may be able to eat those foods often or in large amounts and burn them.

Your metabolism is smaller, weaker and finer. It does a good job running your body on healthy foods. It is meant to keep you healthy. Your metabolism can only handle lower calorie meals. It can only handle the occasional high-calorie treat. It needs fewer calories that you have been giving it.

In a quest to be healthy and happy, you have been feeding it too much. Your subconscious mind always wants what's best for you. Somewhere along the line it picked up the idea you needed large amounts of food to be healthiest. That is wrong. You can throw out that idea forever.

From now on your subconscious mind will realize you require far fewer calories. You enjoy lighter meals. You know you should have smaller portion sizes. That is all your body requires to get all the nutrients it needs and be at its most healthy.

Eating whatever you want to, whenever you want to and as much as you want to, is the wrong answer for your body and for your health.

You are healthiest and feel your best when you are watching your calories. Limiting your portion sizes and eating whole fresh foods. Fruits and vegetables taste wonderful, refreshing and full of life. You feel your healthiest and best when eating light.

(Repeat your RMR Magic Number)

More and more you find yourself focusing on fresh fruits and vegetables and drinking plenty of water. You focus on small servings of lean proteins. You try to keep carbs to a minimum.

SKINNY SECRET 5: SUGAR IS ADDICTIVE

Did you know there has been recent research that found some heavily processed foods are actually addictive and were likely specifically created to be as irresistible as possible by the companies that make them? The phenomenon is known as foods being hyper-palatable and it was publicized by food scientist Steven Witherly. He wrote the book, literally, on "Why Humans Like Junk Food."

You see, in the past foods were either mainly fatty, salty, sour or sweet. Fruits, meats, fats and regular baked goods offered a normal amount of "reward" to your brain for eating them. Nowadays certain highly processed foods are engineered to hit those reward centers so much harder. Many of today's manufacturers have overloaded their products with so much extra sugar, fat and artificial flavoring that they are able to hit your brain's reward centers at a much more extreme level, thus making them addictive. Also, some foods are able to balance all of those flavors so well that no single flavor overpowers any other. That means no flavor really stands out in your mind after you've just eaten and this leaves you longing to eat some more.

One food that does this particularly well is Doritos. Not only are they hyper-palatable, with perfectly balance flavors, they're also engineered to melt in your mouth. They melt so well since half the calories of Doritos come from fat. This leads you to feel, as it melts, that the calories have melted down too. This has been shown to cause you to underestimate the amount of calories you've really eaten. Along with heavily processed foods, when sugar is more than 10% of your diet, it too can become addicting.

Considering that one cup of certain yogurt brands has the same amount of sugar as a glazed doughnut, it's not an exaggeration to say that there is sugar in darn near everything we eat. It's in our bread, our ketchup, in our cereals. This is a problem because sugar causes Dopamine to be released in our brain. When you eat tons of sugar, it then causes tons of dopamine to be released in the brain.

Over time, if we do this a lot, for self-protection some of your body's dopamine receptors start to go away. That means it now takes extra sugar to get the same mental reward, as you used to get when eating just a little sugar. This is very similar to how addicts build up resistance to alcohol or certain drugs, needing more and more of them to get the same kind of high. Now it all makes sense, no wonder some people are eating two candy bars or half a box of cookies in one sitting. That's just what it takes to satisfy them since they're addicted to sugar.

Both sugar and many highly processed foods are hijacking the chemicals in our brains causing us to over eat. These scientific realities are at the heart our country's weight epidemic. The sad thing is that many people don't understand these simple scientific truths. So instead of doing what will work, eating whatever they want as long as it's non-addictive, they spend tons of money on crazy diets that don't work long term. Diets that don't even touch on treating the real reasons they're overweight in the first place. The worst offenders are many of the low-fat and gluten-free products. Often to get rid of extra fat, the low-fat products add extra sugar. Even worse, many of the gluten free products replace the gluten by adding both extra sugar and extra fat.

BREAK THE ADDICTION: FIND JUNK FOOD'S WEAKNESS

What I am about to share with you is my equivalent to McDonald's secret sauce. It is my quickest, easiest and one of my most effective methods for helping someone gain control over their cravings. It gives someone who once would down 8 cookies, 3 big slices of pizza or whatever the case might be, the ability to stop after just a few bites. You know what it is? Helping their mind realize something that is already true, that most people just never fully pick up on. The huge truth is a simple one. As we age, our sense of taste just like our eyesight or our hearing begins to get weaker and weaker. Most adults, if they really took the time to notice or were able to try their trigger foods for the first time, would find that most of them are bland. It really is that simple.

Bread, potatoes and pasta to most adults are nearly tasteless. For many of us grown-ups, if we really take the time to notice it even ice cream suffers from the same problem. Many of us remember it as the sweet vivid treat from our childhood, where the flavor selection had serious importance. Now, if you're really paying attention, as an adult it only tastes sweet, cold and vaguely creamy. If you blindfolded us many of us would have trouble picking out the difference between anything more than the simplest flavors. Pastry like cookies and cakes, acts a lot like bread, the flavor is so bland that in most cases it's just a vaguely sweet floury taste. When eating chips and French fries, most of the time we only taste the grease and the salt (or any added artificial flavoring.) Even with pizza it's the grease and the toppings we taste, not the crust. Sadly, over time, even chocolate for us becomes blander, with just a vague kind of chocolaty sweetness.

Numerous scientific findings have proven time and time again that this is a medical fact. However, it's one thing to intellectually know that your sense of taste has changed. It is another to have your brain specifically tuned into that change, noticing it and really internalizing the truth of what has occurred. Telling people things they know are lies in hypnosis just isn't very effective at creating long-term change, in some cases it can even be disruptive to their staying in hypnosis. That's why my secret sauce, the technique I use to almost instantly give someone more control over their eating, is the simple process of telling them, while in hypnosis, that fruits and veggies have a strong enough flavor to still taste vibrant, appealing and life-giving, while also letting them know that from now on they will begin to notice just how truly bland, greasy and unappealing many of their trigger foods are. It works because it is 100 percent true. Almost everyone eats with their eyes first and their memories second. By the time the food gets to their mouth, they are already mentally tasting it. They are expecting a very specific taste and when they get some of that taste, they chew and move on to the next bite. For most people the fact that their food is getting slightly blander year after year typically goes un-noticed.

HOW TO RE-PROGRAM YOURSELF

Hypnosis, much like meditation, is in part just an accelerated form of learning. It helps you relax, allowing everything else to begin to drop away, even as your mind wanders the rest of the world is shut out. You can suggest to yourself that you will begin to notice that your tastes have changed and that old trigger foods like bread, cakes and cookies are now blander. Suddenly you'll be more attuned to that fact. You don't even have to mentally remember to notice it; your mind will pick up on it more and more. There is one important point to note, though. If you experience this type of habit control only once you may notice a difference as you eat over the next several days or for some individuals even up to two weeks. However, for most people the effect wears off. The reason why? The other worries of life eventually begin to distract them and the way they've always experienced those foods in the past is still part of their memory. Hypnosis is good at creating new memories; it's bad at removing old memories. Therefore, it takes repetition to make the results stick. You have to hear the suggestions and/or imagine the trigger foods as bland over and over again. This keeps the real truth that your tastes really have changed over time at the very front of your mind. You notice that certain foods really, truly have become blander. Do that enough and it becomes your new reality. Once your trigger foods really are blander to you, you really will have more control over how much of them you eat.

BREAK THE HABIT

In the past, when clients came to see us looking to stop smoking not only did we hypnotize them to quit by using suggestions like, "you will feel better not smoking" "cigarettes taste bitter" and "your lungs are getting healthier and healthier each day you go without a cigarette," but we would also give them a habit control schedule. The schedule is a log sheet they fill out showing the times of day they smoke and how much they enjoy each cigarette. Depending on their situation we usually had them continue smoking as they normally did for the first week. Then, we asked them to look at all those times when they smoked and see which cigarettes they most "need" psychologically and which ones they could eliminate with little stress. Some found they smoked about 20 times a day and the cigarette they had during their break at work really helped them feel like they got some down time, but the cigarette first thing in the morning was just more of a habit but not as enjoyable. During their next session we would then ask them to pick the five cigarettes they could fairly easily eliminate each day. Maybe one of them would be that cigarette first thing in the morning that they didn't really enjoy as much. The next week they were again asked to pick five more cigarettes to eliminate, and that continued on and on until they were completely smoke free. This method of habit control is also every effective for weight loss situations and translates exactly as you would expect. Someone hoping to lose a few pounds should eat normally for a week cataloging all the sugar they're eating. They would also be asked to rate how satisfying those foods were to them.

SKINNY SECRET 6: FOOD COMPANIES PLAY MENTAL GAMES

The lies at supermarkets aren't exactly a secret anymore, but they are so sneaky and so common they still fool some of the savviest shoppers. From bags of chips and cookies that look like they should be one serving size but are really 2.5 servings, to deadly trans-fats hiding in your frosting, it's a minefield for your health. Don't you just love the cereal that proudly announces in big lettering that its first ingredient is whole grain? Many of them are hoping no one ever turns the box around to read the fine print on the label showing that sugar is the second largest ingredient. Low calorie cookies are also really great...NOT! Most are so unsatisfying you'll be driven to eat the entire box in a day or two but rationalize, "It was low-fat."

Nearly all the middle aisles of every store are full of marketing gimmicks designed to play into the latest health fad, let you think you are being healthy and get you to pay a premium. Think breakfast cookies, need I say more? Worse yet, with all these promises of healthy options, what they are likely really selling you is the same cheap processed corn, corn syrup, sugar, bleached flour filled trash you have probably already been buying for years. Why don't they want to provide better products with only quality ingredients? There are two reasons. First, corn, corn syrup, white refined flour, fillers and sugar taste great and they are cheap. Since this junk tastes great, companies figure you'll buy the stuff and, secondly, since it's cheap, they get to make the biggest possible profit. It's a win, win for them. The only loser is you, your waistline and your health. Your health, or lack thereof, isn't keeping them up at night. (Unless it is how to better fool you into thinking their sugar, white flour, preservative and salt filled product is actually healthy.)

With family in the fast food business, we probably should leave both fast food and restaurants in general alone. But, we're not. At one point, we even considered opening our own restaurant, continuing a family tradition. We went to all the big food vendor shows, met with their sales people and even tasted all the food. What is scary is that we learned the less chicken they put in the "chicken" the cheaper it is. For example, real white meat chicken chunks are very expensive. White and dark meat chicken chunks are still pretty pricey. But, what is basically chicken mush and fillers pressed and molded into cubes, are much cheaper. Chicken patties and nearly everything else work off that same principle. So the fact is, when you order chicken at many fast food establishments, you are actually eating chicken mush! The ground beef isn't much better. In fact, at certain "value" fast food spots only a certain percentage of the ground beef is actually even real ground beef. Talk about a clear case of getting what you pay for! The rest of most of those super cheap meals are full of white flour, potatoes and, of course, sugar which some places add to almost every item on their menu to make sure it all tastes good. Even more disgusting, almost every fast food place around recycles their fryer oil. It is too expensive to change it daily. Instead, it is filtered to remove the larger old food particles and the fake processed cheese.

In short, there is a reason certain fast food restaurants have a 99 cent menu. The food is cheap, made of cheap poor quality ingredients, which in most cases aren't great for your body. Now to be fair, some fast food places do offer more quality food with more quality ingredients. Here is a hint; it is not on the value menu, unless it's chili. These better-for-you items will usually run you 5 dollars or more, with no fries and a drink. Another example of getting what you pay for.

FIGHT FAST FOOD ADDITION: HARNESS THE GAG REFLEX

Everyone has that one food or that one type of alcohol that they used to love. I want you to remember that one thing that used to just slide down your throat; that used to make you feel so good; that one thing that eventually made you so violently sick that it made you vomit. It might be from food poisoning or too much alcohol.

Remember how sick you were and how just the thought of it now, turns your stomach. I want you to remember how it smells, how just the slightest whiff of it now makes you remember the acidic taste of throwing up. How the very idea of having it sitting in your mouth makes you want to gag. Why is this memory so effective at keeping you from having the food or drink that made you violently ill? You have naturally hypnotized your own subconscious, using that dramatic event, and now naturally avoid consuming as much of that thing that you used to enjoy.

I want you now to imagine your favorite fast food, that one kind of junk food you can't seem to resist. It can be French fries, pizza, cookies, Coca-Cola or a cheeseburger. Whatever it is pick just one. That image will become very clear in your mind. You can remember how it smells. How it feels to hold it in your hands. What it looks like just before you are about to eat it. How it tastes the moment after you put it in your mouth. That image is becoming stronger and stronger. You experience how it would feel in your mouth as you start to chew or swallow. Now I want you to visualize or imagine that first item. That first food or drink that you used to love but now can't stand. How sick you were. How just its smell makes you remember the acidic taste of throwing up. How tasting it makes you want to get it out of your mouth as fast as possible. Visualize that. What does that visual look like? Are you close or are you far away? What is the expression on your face? How is the lighting--is it dim or bright? Where are you with this in your mouth, wanting to spit it out? Really feel that feeling.

Now imagine your favorite fast food in exactly that same way. You are in the same location with the same feeling in the pit of your stomach and with that same expression on your face. The lighting is the same and you have the same taste in your mouth with the same urge to spit it out. This hypnosis is called Neuro Linguistic Programming or NLP for short. It works on an unconscious level and is about understanding how your mind uses light and dark, perspective and feeling to create your associations about certain things. If you can change how your mind perceives or classifies a certain food or item, you can, in effect change, your feelings about it and your need to have it.

For example if you became violently ill drinking tequila and now it smells and tastes like vomit to you, you will have trouble enjoying it now at all. Think about how it appears in your mind, what makes it so unattractive now. You can then use that same mental map, or way of thinking, to repeatedly think about something you want to give up, such as cheeseburgers.

SKINNY SECRET 7: YOU CAN'T HATE EXERCISE AND GET FIT

Did you know that only 5% of the population are actually real gym goers? Only 5% of the people we sell a gym membership to will use it on a regular basis, coming in at least 3 to 5 times a week. You may know these people as "gym rats".

We have noticed they think differently and train differently than the other people we see in the gym around January trying to make this year the year they'll really get in shape. Here's what sets the "gym rats" apart. The "gym rats" see the gym as a social destination. They make connections at the gym. They make it fun. They don't come in and kill themselves at the gym every time they pop in for a workout. They only kill themselves with a really hard work out when they feel like it. When they are enjoying pushing themselves and want to celebrate what their body is capable of.

Much of the time, we see our "gym rats" spending a lot of their time chatting. They chat with us, they chat with the manager and they chat with each other. The gym is a place where they have friends and they enjoy coming in. They taught us if you want long term success it has be enjoyable. Not torture! In a word, don't sign up for a butt-kicking boot camp, unless that is the kind of thing you really enjoy. One of my favorite "gym rats" works out nearly every day and has been an avid exerciser ever since high school. She loves taking time out for herself. She enjoys having a fit trim body that she's proud off. She often works out with friends. She loves to try new classes. She really enjoys them and finds them fun and doesn't seem to have any fears about embarrassing herself by falling behind the group or doing a move wrong. She has good "work out self-esteem." The reason she loves going to the gym is that it gives her a chance to try new things and because it gives her a toned body that makes her feel really good about herself. Sometimes she goes to the gym and really makes herself sweat, probably imagining much of the time how great her butt is going to look in her jeans and how great being in shape makes her look. Other times she goes to the gym and does a light to moderate workout because she's chatting and really enjoying herself. Everyone has to find exactly what works for them. It's important to discover which of the many possible motivating factors out there most inspires you. It doesn't have to be joining a gym. Maybe you would like to jog with a friend, take dance lessons or go hiking.

WHY WE HATE EXERCISE

Imagine a child who is always picked last for teams, the heavy kid who runs a 14 minute mile and finishes dead last gasping for breath or the scrawny boy who can't do a single pull up just hanging there in front of the whole class. These types of kids had bad experiences with exercise, often repeatedly. They are likely to tell themselves, "I'm just not very athletic", "I hate PE", "I am not good at running", or "I don't like to sweat". They may even feel panic at the idea of facing a PE class, picking teams or working out.

These are feelings that often don't go away with age, making these kids more likely to lead a sedentary lifestyle as adults. These grownups then use excuses like, "I just don't have time to exercise" or "It's just too miserable," and so they never manage to get into a long-term fitness routine. Even people who were once former athletes and had good experiences with physical activity early on can fall into this trap.

Growing up they may have seen parents who didn't exercise or who at least put a higher value on other things. They perhaps valued job success or family time more than making it a point to maintain their health. These values are often unconsciously conveyed and kids tend to unintentionally mimic what they see. Still, when they fail to lose weight most people don't blame their programming but instead blame themselves over and over again.

They don't understand about their subconscious and how it impacts their decision-making, and instead believe their conscious mind is completely in control when, really, it's only responsible for a small part of their behavior.

HOW TO START TO LOVE EXERCISE

You can imagine yourself walking, running or working out and really enjoying it. You feel at peace. You feel good about yourself and the time you are taking to work on your body. This is something you give yourself, so you can be your best. You find you are happiest when you are exercising and moving more. These are the types of messages you'll want to give yourself. Eventually, when you feel positive enough, you can begin to go walking or head to the local gym. Just make sure you keep telling yourself the positive message and make sure that each experience is very positive and comfortable.

EXERCISE HYPNOSIS

In hypnosis, imagine yourself back in PE class. This time though you are feeling strong, confident and accepted. You have a new teacher. Visualize or imagine what she looks like and how they sound. They sit the entire class down on some soft grass and start to explain to them and to you how the human body works. They explain that aerobic exercise not only burns calories, it expands lung capacity. The teacher then tells the class that people who smoke can develop COPD because they have damaged their lungs and once their lungs aren't functioning properly their hearts have to work harder and harder. That is what leads to many smokers dying from heart attacks before lung cancer ever becomes a factor. Lung capacity is very important to long-term health for non-smokers, too, and that is what we increase every time we do aerobic activity.

The new PE teacher goes on to explain that to prevent most cases of diabetes, heart attacks and stroke you only need 30 minutes of moderate walking 5 days a week. She then has the entire class stand up and walk onto a large dirt track. She has everyone, including you, take 4 steps. "Now you are all walkers," she says. She then has everyone run a very short distance. "Stop, Stop. I want you to know you are now all runners, that is all it takes" she explains. With a smile on her face she says, "If you walk, you are a walker. If you jog, you are a jogger. If you run, no matter how slowly, you are a runner. Best of all, if you are doing something athletic, you are an athlete."

Now she has everyone begin to run around the track and with every step she shouts to them, "You are saving your own life. You are expanding your lung capacity; you are helping your heart. You are keeping yourself healthy with every step you take." Now she has everyone chanting it, "With every step I take I am saving my own life. I am rescuing myself from heart disease, high blood pressure and diabetes." Yelling it now, cheering it now, with their arms in the air, "I am saving my own life with every step I take!" Be your own cheerleader now as you start your exercise program.

MENTAL SECRET 8: MAKE EVERYDAY A CHEAT DAY

A lot of people have trouble sticking perfectly to a diet for a long period without cheating. In fact, most thin people give themselves a treat now and then. Almost everyone does at some time, at least once a week. That brings us to the option of making every day a cheat day, where you are allowed to eat anything you want to, without feeling any guilt or having it impact your dieting in any way. The bonus to using this method is that it makes cheating a planned event, something you can look forward to.

This is also a great method for people who have emotional issues tied to junk food. Where, for example, sweets which are seen as "forbidden" are, therefore, irresistible and bring with them a great deal of shame after they are eaten. People often denied certain foods as children, or shamed by their parents for eating sweets, fall into this trap. Planning to cheat can give you permission to eat what you want; lessening the control those foods have over you. It can also help you resolve feelings of guilt related to eating junk food. When the guilt goes away and no food is ever completely forbidden, those foods then lose that feeling of being irresistible. In short, "cheating" helps put you back in control of your eating. Obviously there is a major downside of too much cheating, as it does slow down the weight loss process. You'll want to make sure you watch your portion sizes. Not only does this planned cheating taste great, it can make it even easier to make sure you stick with it and succeed... for the rest of your life! My secret is hypnosis. You can eat whatever you want just as long as you are in control of your cravings. I do that for my clients in two ways. First, I get them physically unaddicted then I get them mentally unaddicted. Let me explain.

BACK SLIDING

Many people try to be perfect when on a diet and then when they cheat feel that all is lost and will blow that diet completely, sometimes for days or weeks, sometimes even longer. The exact opposite is really the true. Backsliding or resistance is often a good sign. It shows that you have been making progress and are leveling off a bit. You level off a bit and then you will start making progress again. It is completely natural to feel some resistance when you are trying to make a major life change. Some people may even gain a few pounds at one point as their body and mind resist turning a brand new corner in their life.

Our bodies naturally resist change and, generally, it takes a good deal of effort to shift weight up or down. Doing what we have always done makes us feel safe and comfortable. The unknown is stress provoking and scary. You have experienced the phenomenon known as resistance anytime you have moved to a new city, changed jobs or gone to a new school. Your heart races, you are afraid of the unknown, nervous about what might happen and about not fitting in. Many people find themselves thinking, "This isn't the way my old neighborhood was," or "This isn't how we did things at my old job or school." Part of them often wants to go back to their old city, school or job.

This resistance is normal and it is always part of growing and moving forward in your life. Recognizing that a major shift in the way you eat, exercise and think is also a significant life change is important. You should expect resistance and diet slip-ups as part of the process of lasting change. Release any guilt and move on.

DIAL BACK THE CRAVINGS HYPNOSIS

I want you to imagine yourself at a place of deepest temptation for you. It could be in front of the refrigerator, or during a certain holiday or perhaps visiting family or even a certain restaurant. It is ok to pick just one.

I want you to imagine this place of greatest temptation, where everything looks tempting and your resolve to eat small amounts of healthy food seems to almost vanish. Perhaps it's habit, or just that the foods there are very tempting or foods that you don't often have access to.

Today we are going to work on a technique to gain back control using numbers. Your subconscious mind easily understands numbers.

First, I want you to mentally picture in your mind those various foods you would expect to see in this very tempting situation.

From now on you will have a new tool. I want you to picture a dial on your chest with numbers from 0 to 10. Zero means you don't want anything. Ten means the craving for junk food is nearly uncontrollable. From now on you will only give in and satisfy your craving or the desire to snack if the dial is at a 9 or above. Let me repeat that...*only* if the dial is at a 9 or above.

Now let's practice. I want you to think of one food item you would likely encounter in this place of greatest temptation. You notice the dial on your chest and all the food surrounding you. If the dial is at a 5, or 6, from now on you will ignore it. A 5 or a 6 means this is a craving you should ignore. It will likely pass. When you have a craving that is a 5 or a 6 you get something to drink. Perhaps flavored water, peppermint tea or any low-calorie warm drink. From now on when a craving is only a 5 or a 6 you will know what to do. You will get a something to drink. It will satisfy that craving.

Now picture another food. Something you would crave at a 7 or 8. What does a 7 or 8 mean? You see the food sitting there or can imagine eating it. It seems to be calling to you. You get something to drink and find something else that needs your attention. You distract yourself for 30 minutes. Thirty minutes is the magic number.

If the dial is at a 9 or 10, you have a small amount of the

item you are craving.

From now on, nothing is off limits. Every food is ok in moderation. Moderation is the key to life-long weight loss. Moderation is part of the lifestyle you will adopt.

From now on, if the dial is at a 9 or 10 you will have a small amount of the item you were craving.

SKINNY SECRET 9: GET MORE SLEEP AND STRESS LESS

There are a million studies all over the internet, in almost every woman's magazine, next to the supermarket cash register and quoted in nearly every weight loss book at Barnes and Noble. Some are worthwhile, others are obvious and others may make you wonder why they were ever studied at all. The best study I've heard of is the Sleep-Stress Secret. I have found it proven true time and time again, not only in my own life but with hundreds of my clients as well. What researchers have discovered is that weight loss isn't about how much willpower you have. It isn't about your strength of mind.

It's about where the rubber meets the road on a daily basis and that involves two factors. Those two factors are the amount of sleep you've gotten and the amount of stress you're currently under. To put it another way, if you have zero energy and are finding it a struggle to just get through the day, then you are being forced to put your focus on mundane tasks and simple survival, what you're not focusing on is sticking to your plan to lose weight. You're desperate, you're tired and you're probably eating something you shouldn't just to get some energy to get through the day. The other major factor is stress. Or, to put it another way, if you are feeling worried, sad, upset or angry you will be focusing on that emotion, thinking about the circumstances around what has you upset and possible focusing your energy on what you are going to about this problem in the future or obsessing about how it could possibly get worse.

One guess what you're not thinking about. If you guessed losing weight and choosing healthy foods in the right amounts, you guessed right! Even worse, if you're an emotional eater, you may even be mindlessly shoveling large amounts of comfort foods into your mouth while barely noticing exactly what or how much you're eating. Knowing about the Sleep-Stress secret is a powerful weight loss tool. If you can get enough sleep and work to keep yourself on a pretty even keel emotionally that half the battle is already won. Set yourself a nightly sleep goal and explore coping techniques that will help you relax—for example reading, listening to music or meditating.

SKINNY SECRET 10: YOUR MEMORIES ARE KEEPING WEIGHT ON

Despite our best intentions when it comes to dieting at some time or another we are all our own worst enemy. We have all held ourselves back, sabotaged our own success and fallen victim to our own bad habits. This universal experience of struggling to lose weight, eat healthily and move more can best be explained by the idea that comes from the psychological theory, known as the "Theory of Mind."

The "Theory of Mind" states that until about age 10 we learn about the world and create what become our automatic ideas about the world around us. It's the basic stuff that controls the way we think, what things we think are good and what things we think are bad. For example, if your grandma bakes cookies every summer, in all your favorite flavors, just for you and being with her is when you feel deeply loved, then you will have great memories linked to those cookies. Those cookies will be more than just simple cookies to you; they will mean love, comfort, and security. Therefore, with those great associations, her cookies and likely all homemade cookies, in general, will be nearly impossible to resist. Whether it's that favorite cake you always got on your birthday or a favorite meal your family prepared for celebrations, there are certain foods we become addicted to that mean a lot more to us than just satisfying hunger or giving us a sugar rush.

If your family used desserts or junk food as a reward, a celebration, a way to unwind, a way to soothe away hurts or a way to bond, those foods become part of who you are. Cake might become your way to celebrate, your comfort food, your way to deal with stress and chocolate may become your way to treat yourself. So now, even as an adult when you want to celebrate a holiday, cope with stress or just take a mental vacation, if you aren't consciously thinking about it, you'll reach for the cake, the chocolate, the chips, the ice cream, the cookies or something else that will make the pounds pile on.

EXACTLY HOW IT HAPPENS

This is the "secret recipe" to raise a child that will likely struggle with weight issues for the rest of their lives. It is not only written as an example of what not to do. It is also written so that when you read this you can identify certain factors from your own childhood that may be contributing to your struggles with weight. To create someone who will likely have weight issues, first create a lot of great positive memories centering around unhealthy foods. You want to make sure family celebrations, birthdays, and holidays have food as a major focus. Picture decadent family dinners, glorious birthday cakes and plates piled high with an assortment of cookies and candies. The trick to creating that strong positive association is to make sure the good feelings are flowing and the unhealthy foods are front and center.

It's also best to have especially loving one on one time with a child while the food is present and use certain treats to mark every special occasion. Second, once the child has a strong love for certain junk foods, make sure to limit those drastically creating feelings of scarcity. Give the candy and snacks freely during holidays and other celebrations, then randomly take them away at other times with little explanation. If your child sneaks it or eats it during those times make sure they know that's bad and they should feel guilty and shameful. Making certain treats forbidden and somewhat naughty works wonders at strengthening an almost addiction like love of those foods. They become forbidden and so are nearly irresistible.

Next, it's important to employ what psychology calls the Pain Pleasure Principle. Humans feel pleasure doing what is known to them and pain at facing the unknown. That's why, if your goal is to raise a fat child, try to make sure a diet high in healthy foods like fruits and vegetables is completely foreign to them. Get them used to a diet high in meat, dairy, fat and carbohydrates, so that's what they will be most comfortable with. It's also important to have them eat only three times a day or less since eating many smaller meals throughout the day can help lead to weight loss. It's far better to make sure there is a giant sized main meal late in the day. At that meal, they will likely overeat and make poor food choices since they are so hungry. It also helps if you force them to clean their plate, that way they get used to overeating and form strong negative associations with any healthy foods they are forced to eat. It's like killing two birds with one stone. Also, make sure they get used to having dessert every night. It's a great habit to form, that can help them avoid weight loss for life.

Next it's on to exercise. Make sure to do as little outdoor activity with your kids as possible. Playing catch, kicking the soccer ball around or going for a pleasant walk around the neighborhood will only encourage them to like these healthy activities. If you must be active with them, make sure it's a negative experience, filled with high expectations, yelling and disappointed looks.

Finally, make sure there are plenty of great indoor sedentary options for the child to do. We want video games, movies, and hours of TV to the main form of daily entertainment. This will likely become a habit they can continue well into adulthood and with maintain for life.

Congratulations, if you do all this you too can raise a child with bad eating habits and a hatred for exercise. Give it time and you'll see that you have successfully created a child that is nearly certain to eventually be overweight. Or you can do the exact opposite of these instructions and raise a thin healthy person!

HOW TO FIX IT

Here is the great part, yes; you can reprogram yourself by creating new positive feelings about healthy foods and exercise. We all know that dramatic real-life experiences can change the way we think and behave, often forever. People who suffer a traumatic event often become more fearful of situations that never scared them before. They become fearful and stressed when faced with a similar situation or event. They may even give up some of their favorite activities because of the deep fear that can be created in an instant.

On the flip side, people who are given a huge reward or find unexpected major success can suddenly become more confident. They will attempt things they have never tried before and will feel more empowered to go after large goals. That one experience, good or bad, can often change the course of their entire lives. Here's the interesting thing, the mind can't tell the difference between these real life dramatic events actually happening or just a vivid daydream. Hypnosis is actually just a fancy word for a very common state of trance that we, meaning every person on the planet, put themselves into on an almost daily basis. If you get caught up in a movie, start crying with the main character or get terrified during a scary part, the reality of sitting in a movie theater has dropped away and you have been hypnotized.

Scientists have actually studied how people's brains and bodies respond to trauma. Their brain scans show that the response in the body and the brain are the exact same whether a subject really experiences a situation or just vividly imagines it. Understanding that the mind can't tell the difference between a real event and one that is vividly imagined is one of the major underpinnings of hypnosis. If you can create dramatic events in your mind, you can reprogram how the mind responds to the world.

IMAGINE YOURSELF HAVING A "THIN" UPBRINGING

Sometimes you just want to hate those people who are "naturally thin". Especially when they tell you about how much willpower they have, how mentally strong they think they are or, worse yet, how lazy or self-indulgent they think someone struggling with their weight is.

Still, you can't really blame them. They just don't get it. It's a lot like why a rich kid might not understand how much harder someone who's grown up poor might have to fight to reach their same level of success. A "naturally thin" person doesn't understand the mental road blocks that can spring up for a heavy person trying to lose a few pounds.

The reason those "naturally thin" people often just don't get it, is that their unconscious is working for them. They generally see exercise as a way to make their bodies strong and maintain their health. They may have good, strong memories of playing outside with their parents or working out as a family. Exercise was likely important in their home, so when they exercise they feel pride in doing something good for themselves, instead of panic. They see working out as an important priority and don't dread exercise or feel as if it's a waste of their time.

When it comes to food "naturally thin" people may have great healthy memories of watermelon in the summertime, plates of brightly colored fruits, sweet potatoes at Grandma's and hot buttered corn on summer vacation. They have fewer strong emotional memories tied to junk food and more strong emotional memories involving healthier choices and smaller portions. It's also more likely that their families didn't use unhealthy foods as a reward, as an emotional Band-Aid or as a way to bond.

They likely got access to sweets when they wanted them, no one ever made a very big deal about junk food and most meals were fairly low calorie; featuring fruits, veggies, and lean meats. The "good" food wasn't gross and they have lots of great memories involving low-cal summery foods. With hypnosis... you can too.

JUST FAKE IT

Love keeps us fat. In fact, love has been helping you get fat and stay fat for a long time. How you ask is love making us fat? Here's how... your mom loved you and made birthday cakes on your birthday, made a special effort to bake Christmas cookies with you at Christmas time, your Grandma loved you so much she made all your favorite "treat" foods whenever you visited, your family loved you so much they celebrated every holiday with a huge family feast, your honey gets all of your favorite fast foods or pizza for special movie or TV show nights. Sadly, all those good memories tend for most of us to add up to extra inches and pounds.

Why, you ask? Because, those moments are unforgettable! They are some of the best, richest and more meaningful moments in our lives. They are often some of our happiest memories, so good we want to relive them over and over again. Even though those times have past, we recreate the feelings for ourselves with the foods that bring back those memories. We tend to celebrate the way we've always celebrated. Love our kids with the same traditions our parents gave us, Christmas cookies included. The same heavy recipes are used over and over, because it's tradition, because of the memories they instantly bring to the surface the moment you taste or smell them.

This is one of the hardest issues to overcome, even for weight loss hypnotists. Many just stop at helping people find trigger foods less attractive or work on portion sizes, ignoring this massive piece of the puzzle. I guess they just can't find a creative way to battle unforgettable memories, often the best of our lives, which are centered directly around food. You can't just tell someone that they don't matter to them anymore. Their mind, including their subconscious, would just reject that as a lie, making it ineffective long term.

Here is the solution… hypnosis is great for creating false memories. It's so good many courts consider witnesses tainted after undergoing hypnosis. It's so good Freud accidentally used it to convince a bunch of his female patients they'd been molested by their fathers when further investigation proved that to be untrue. I bet you've guessed it. If not, here's another clue. Remember, your mind can't tell the difference between what you vividly imagine and what you actually experience. So here is the answer, in hypnosis or when using self-hypnosis, I recommend focusing on creating new positive, powerful, and unforgettable memories involving much healthier choices.

For the record, one great healthy food memory can't out

weight 20 years of unforgettable memories involving heavy food, cookies, candy and cake. Still, three unforgettable memories involving more positive choices "experienced" (listened to or imagined) over and over again can begin to make an impact. Add in one more element and you'll start to see amazing results. Can you figure it out? Here is your clue, remember those witnesses who get more details right thanks to hypnosis but the court considers those memories are considered tainted because they're afraid he could identify the wrong bad guy. Well, hypnosis can tweak how you remember certain details of actual events that really did happen.

So what is the answer, the secret, the final step to tipping those emotional eating scales? Relive those some of those wonderful holiday dinners, movie nights and Grandma time, but this time mentally remove those unhealthy treats and add in a strong dose of yummy yet healthier choices. Do both these techniques enough and suddenly that seemingly unbreakable bond between certain foods and the positive emotions they create begin to break!

Allison Staley C.Ht. & Ryan Staley C.Ht.

SKINNY SECRET 11: THIN OUT YOUR FAVORITES

Once you get used to having a cheat day, you can begin to take it to the next level. You can start to take that one day a week when you allow yourself to have any and all the foods you love and make it just a little healthier. I like to call this process, "Thinning Out Your Favorites." Taking this one simple step can help make sure that once you lose the weight you keep it off. Start making a few of your favorite recipes a little healthier and you'll save yourself tens of thousands of calories over your lifetime.

For example, eggs get most of their calories from the yolks. An egg is about 90 calories. The yolk is about 75 calories. The egg white is only 15 calories. Egg yolk does have things in it that are beneficial to our health, so it is important to use some of it. When making scrambled eggs, I recommend using 1 egg yolk and 3 egg whites. You can even mix in a little low-fat cottage cheese to make the eggs creamy. They'll be the right color, taste nearly as good and be far easier on your waistline.

Many people just can't seem to give up pasta, although it is one of the most calorie dense foods you could possibly eat. The solution for many may be to find a healthier substitute for regular pasta, such as Shirataki noodles. They are traditional Japanese noodles made from a yam. They can be found in many health foods stores or in the refrigerated health food aisle of certain grocery stores. They have almost no carbohydrates and have very few calories. They can be eaten as the only pasta in a dish or they can be mixed with traditional pasta to lighten the meal up.

You can also lighten up most of the store bought mixes for cakes, cupcakes, bread and brownies by using Greek yogurt. You simply substitute one cup of Greek yogurt and one cup of water for the eggs and oil you would usually add to the recipe. Often you can barely tell the difference and you have cut out tons of fat and calories. In the fall, instead of using Greek yogurt, you can also use a small can of pumpkin.

You can also substitute Greek yogurt for butter in many

recipes and it works to lighten heavy dips and sauces because it can stand in for a certain amount of cream and cheese.

RECIPES

Amazing Banana Waffles

¼ cup   Old-Fashioned Oatmeal (ground)

7-9   Egg Whites

3 tbsp.   Splenda Sugar Substitute

½ tsp.   Cinnamon

½ tsp.   Vanilla Extract

½   Mashed Banana

Directions:

1. Mix all ingredients together by hand.

2. Pour serving sizes into a greased waffle maker.

3. Cook each waffle until golden brown.

RECIPES

Raisin Cinnamon Oatmeal

¼ cup Old-Fashioned Oatmeal (ground)

¼ cup Greek Yogurt

3 tbsp. Splenda Sugar Substitute

½ tsp. Cinnamon

¼ cup Vanilla Almond Milk

20 Raisins

Directions:

1. Mix all ingredients together by hand.

2. Pour into an air tight container.

3. Let sit overnight inside the refrigerator. Serve.

RECIPES

Extra Creamy Scrambled Eggs

1   Whole Egg

4   Egg Whites

1   Cottage Cheese
tbsp.

½   Mrs. Dash Seasoning
tsp.

2   Diced Red Pepper
tbsp.

2   Diced Onion
tbsp.

Directions:

1. Mix all ingredients, except seasoning, together by hand.

2. Pour into a hot, greased frying pan and scramble.

3. Sprinkle with Mrs. Dash. Serve.

RECIPES

Sweet Berry Smoothie

¼ cup   Vanilla Almond Milk

¼ cup   Frozen Blueberries

3 tbsp.   Creamy Vanilla Yogurt

3-4   Frozen Strawberries

½ tsp.   Stevia Natural Sweetener

Directions:

1. Mix all ingredients together in a blender.

2. Add ice or water to reach desired texture.

3. Serve and enjoy.

RECIPES

Peanut Butter Bars

¼ cup	Ground Flax Seed
1 can	Garbanzo Beans (drained, rinsed & ground)
1 cup	Splenda Sugar Substitute
½ cup	Peanut Butter
2 tsp.	Vanilla Extract
1 cup	Chopped Peanuts
¼ tsp.	Baking Soda & Baking Powder (1/4 tsp. each)
1	Egg

Directions:

1. Preheat oven to 350 degrees. Bake bars in an 8x8 greased pan for 25-30 minutes.

RECIPES

Guilt Free Alfredo

8 tbsp.	Reduced-Fat Grated Parmesan
4 wedges	Laughing cow Light Swiss Cheese Spread
4 tsp.	Fat-Free Sour Cream
1 pinch	Salt
1 pinch	Pepper

Directions:

1. Mix all ingredients together with a hand mixer.

2. Pour over whole wheat or tofu shirataki noodles.

3. Serve. (Consider adding broccoli and/or grilled chicken.)

RECIPES

Easy Egg Salad

¼ cup   Greek Yogurt

7-9   Egg Whites (coarsely chopped)

2   Whole Eggs

1 pinch   Salt

1 pinch   Pepper

1 tsp.   Mustard

Directions:

1. Hard boil eggs and remove shells.

2. Mix ingredients together. (Optional: add 2 tbsp. chopped pickle or relish.)

3. Serve on salad or whole wheat bread.

RECIPES

Decadent Pumpkin Date Muffins

1 pkg   Krusteaz Oat Bran Muffin Mix

¾ cup   Water

½ cup   Canned Ground Pumpkin

½ cup   Chopped Dates

1½ tsp.   Pumpkin Pie Spice

Directions:

1. Mix all ingredients together by hand.

2. Bake at 400 degrees for 18-20 minutes.

3. Cook until slightly browned.

RECIPES

Better For You Brownies

1 pkg   Betty Crocker (Regular or Low Fat) Fudge Brownie Mix

2   Whole Eggs

¼ cup   Water

½ cup   Plain or Greek Non-Fat Yogurt

.

Directions:

1. Mix all ingredients together by hand.

2. Bake at 350 degrees for roughly 25 minutes.

3. Cook until baked through.

RECIPES

Fresh Cranberry Relish

1 Small Orange

1 12-Ounce Bag Fresh Cranberries (rinsed)

½ cup Chopped Walnuts

¾ cup Stevia or Splenda Sugar Substitute

.

Directions:

1. Grate orange rind and chopped remaining orange into chunks.

2. Put cranberries and orange pieces into food chopper and blend until fine.

3. Mix orange rind, chopped fruit mix, walnuts and sugar substitute together by hand. Chill and serve.

RECIPES

Apple Cranberry Muffins

1 pkg   Krusteaz Fat Free Apple Cinnamon Muffin
Mix

1 cup   Water

¾
cup   Fresh Cranberry Relish

Directions:

1. Mix all ingredients together by hand.

2. Bake at 400 degrees for 18-20 minutes.

3. Cook until slightly browned.

SKINNY SECRET 12: GUZZLING WATER MAKES WEIGHT LOSS EASY

I want to share a sneaky way you can burn more calories by ADDING something to your Diet. Now it's not a milkshake, Coca-Cola, or even frozen yogurt, but it is ICE COLD. This wonderful addition is ICE COLD (33-degree) WATER!!! The principle is simple… your body maintains a constant 98.6 degrees. When you introduce 33-degree water, your body must BURN calories to heat that water up. Water contains exactly ZERO calories. It has been calculated that the average person requires 17.5 calories to heat up a 16 oz glass of ICE COLD water(**). This means by adding THREE 16 oz glasses of ICE COLD water… you have just zapped 50 calories! You MUST incorporate three ICE COLD 16 oz glasses of water per day…. It couldn't be easier!

In fact, please drink your THREE 16 oz glasses of water before eating a meal, having one before breakfast, one before lunch and one before dinner. This habit alone can help you drop up to 5 pounds. Researchers verified this with a 12-week study of nearly 50 people. All the people in the study were put on a low-calorie diet. The only difference was that that some of the participants were told to drink a glass of water before each meal. The water drinkers lost an average of 4.5 pounds more than the non-water drinkers.

This principle also works on a whole other level to help prevent snacking. Did you know that researchers have proven that dehydration causes the body to start mixing up its signals about hunger? That's right, if you're not drinking enough water your body is likely feeling sluggish and tired. It is sending signals to the brain that you need more energy. Your brain can often interpret these signals to mean that you need food. By not giving your body enough water, you are, in effect, tricking your brain into telling you that you are hungry way too often. If you have dry lips, dry skin, dry eyes or darker yellow urine, this could be happening to you! You can also kick your water up enough by sometimes adding tea to it. It can be White Tea, Rooibos, or Pu-erh Tea. These types of tea have been shown to help get rid of belly fat. Researchers in China specifically studied Pu-erh Tea with amazing results. They had two groups of people eat a high fat diet. The only difference is that they had one group fed different amounts of pu-erh tea extract. Those getting the tea showed lower triglycerides in the blood (the dangerous fat that can clog arteries) and lower belly fat. Drink up!

Don't forget to sip on some Green Tea too, though. It's been shown by researchers to increase fat burning and boost your metabolic rate. In fact, one study of only men showed that the tea alone boosted their body's calorie burning potential by 4%. These effects are likely due, in part, to the caffeine found in green tea, so it's not great right before bed.

SKINNY SECRET 13: IT HELPS TO HAVE FAITH

I am not saying you have to believe in God or anything else to lose weight. My only point in this chapter is to say that, if you do happen to have faith, it can be an incredible source of strength and it will improve your odds of losing the weight and keeping it off.

There have been many different studies done on the power of belief and religion on such things as recovery time from surgery, serious disease and even addiction. When the person had faith and used it as a source of support to help them face any of those major challenges, the final results were generally better. People who relied on their faith when recovering from surgery had a faster and better recovery. People who had faith to lean on when suffering from a major illness tended to have a better chance of overcoming it and regaining their health. People who are battling addiction, who lean on God or their higher power when the cravings hit, tend to have a better chance of beating their addiction. This power of faith to help give people strength and carry them through major struggles is likely one of the reasons God and religion is at the heart of many 12 Step Programs such as Alcoholics Anonymous, Narcotics Anonymous, and Over-Eaters Anonymous.

Many people sometimes feel weak. They feel like they don't have the inner strength, deep down inside, not to devour an entire bag of chips or half a box of cookies. That's where faith comes in. It works! Even in at my own weight loss center we have found faith to help increase our client's odds of achieving their weight loss goals.

The hypnosis technique that follows is my own adaptation of one of the methods I was taught during my training at the Hypnosis Motivation Institute, a nationally accredited school for hypnotherapy. I often use this technique to help my clients, who believe in some type of higher power, better access the strength and support that their faith gives them.

HYPNOSIS FOR THE FAITHFUL

Imagine yourself walking down a wooded path. You can see the dirt on the path; hear it crunching under your feet as you walk. Looking to your left and your right you can see the grass bordering the path. You can see trees off in the distance. Are they Oak or Poplar, Elm or Fir? Notice the different colors of green and how the light shimmers through the leaves. You may even feel a gentle breeze beginning to blow around the top of your head, moving down now around your shoulders and arms.

You continue walking down the path, going further and further down the path. You can even notice if there are any particular smells of nature. Maybe the way it smells after a recent rain or just the fresh smell of nature. Off in the distance you now can see a hint of light shining down on this path. As you continue walking down the path getting closer and closer, you can see the light more and more clearly. It appears to be piercing down through the clouds and forming a pool of light on the path directly in front to you. And you can notice the color of the light, how bright or dim it is and how large of area it is shining down on. As I count from 3 down to 1 you will see yourself walking over to that light and stepping into it. 3...2...1.

Stepping into the light now. You can feel it all around you. Again you notice the color inside the light and you take a moment to really feel what the light is or what is in the light. Is it a healing light? Is there a feeling of calm, peace or love in the light? Taking a moment and noticing what the light is, where you think it is coming from and what you feel in it. And, when you are ready, you can bring the challenges you are currently facing, with food or otherwise, into the light. Explaining your struggles now. And, when you are ready, you can ask this light to help you, give you strength to overcome these challenges. You can ask this light for help.

Give yourself a moment to just feel this light all around you. Open yourself up to it. Is there anything it has to communicate to you? Just listen. Just feel what is in the light. And, in a moment, when you are ready, I am going to have you step out of the light.

Stepping out of the light now, taking with you all of the peace, calm and strength you felt in the light. Taking with you any learning or support. And these feelings will go deeper by the day, deeper by the week and deeper by the month. Coming out now. 1...2...3...4...5

SKINNY SECRET 14: MISERY MAKES US FAT

Did you know that it really is impossible to hypnotize anyone against their will? If someone realizes you are trying to hypnotize them, they can concentrate on staying completely present in the moment and analyze every word you are saying. They can refuse to tune out. They can refuse to relax and let go. They can refuse to let any suggestion sink it. Just like it is impossible to hypnotize anyone who doesn't what to be hypnotized, it is impossible to simply decide that someone needs to lose weight and force them to lose it.

Losing weight has to be your own choice for your own reason. Trying to lose weight because someone else thinks you need to lose the weight typically will be gigantically unsuccessful. The most unsuccessful clients I have had were the ones where someone else heard about my program or saw my ads online and bought them in for a session. I've even had a husband drag his wife in to see me and sign her up. He sat down in my office with her next to him and proceeded to tell me all about her problem with food. She said she wanted to do my program and wanted to lose weight. It was clear; however, she just wanted to lose weight because her husband would like it if she were thinner. I tried to make the program all about her. During her first session, I told her to forget about his thoughts concerning her weight and focus on herself. There was just one major problem thought, she, herself, deep down, was really OK with her weight. She wasn't ready to change and wasn't ready to deny even the slightest impulse to have a treat. The motivation just wasn't there. When someone is dragged in to see me, I can't force them, even with hypnosis, to have that real, long-term, deep down desire to be thin.

People have a host of different things that motivate them deeply, from the shallow desire of simply wanting to look better to having health issues due to their eating habits and wanting to save their own life. Some people can even lose weight because they really want to be healthier or look more attractive for someone else, but those thoughts and feelings are arising from deep down within them.

They are not an idea that someone else has pushed on them.

With hypnosis I can make certain foods appear a bit less attractive or seem bland. I can help people think about stopping eating food way before they normal would stop. I can help someone drink water a bit more often or realize on a deeper level why exercise really is important and shouldn't be their last priority. Using hypnosis, I can even help some people uncover emotions they buried down deep, causing them to eat emotionally and hypnosis can actually help them deal with those emotions directly.

I cannot, and have had no success, in creating the deep down original desire to be thin. I can help strengthen someone's resolve to be thin. I can help people trying to lose weight stay on track. I have had no luck, though, getting someone who really didn't have a problem with their weight within themselves lose weight and keep it off. Bottom line, the desire to be thin has to come from within you. You can't lose weight because someone else thinks you should. You can lose weight because you desire to be thinner yourself, to look better for another person, but you can't lose weight because they desperately think you should. Yes, there is a difference and, yes, that difference matters hugely.

GOING DEEPER: THE BEAST CALLED EMOTIONAL EATING

We can all recognize the beast called emotional eating. Sometimes it starts with just being around your boss, or a bad day for your spouse that then becomes a bad day for you, or stress from the kids or just another go around with that same old issue you've been trying to ignore for months, or even years. It can be a feeling of panic, being overwhelmed, or maybe you're just one of those people who simply get in the "zone." We all know what it's like to be in the "zone" and have been there ourselves more than once in our lives. The "zone" is when food just magically appears in our hand, or the box of cookies on our lap, and we're reaching into it over and over and over again as our eyes glaze over and we stare into space. It can happen after work, after a big fight, from boredom or even just as our way to unwind after dinner each night.

Emotional eating is rooted in pain. It is the most destructive type of eating. When you are eating mindlessly, all of a sudden time passes. You have no idea how much you've eaten, but you do know that half the box of cookies has somehow magically disappeared. You feel stuffed. You feel bloated. Then, you feel bad about yourself for pigging out and downing way more sugar, salt, fat, or carbs than you ever meant to. It happens to us over and over again.

Emotional eating is like being in a trance or on some sort of weird autopilot. You feel out of control, unable to resist and usually wind up feeling even worse about yourself than when you started. It causes a cycle of emotional pain that has even led to full blown depression in some. You feel bad, so you eat, you eat too much and feel worse, you find you're gaining weight and feel bad about yourself, you feel bad about yourself so you eat even more.

The definition of emotional eating is being trapped in a rut, feeling an emotion and heading for food. It becomes automatic, your way to deal with any strong feeling. Most people who are trapped in this cycle barely even notice anymore that they are even having an emotion by the time the food is already in their mouth. Then, once it is they zone out, using food as a distraction and don't think anything else about what they're really feeling. The food does nothing to fix what's causing the emotion; it's just a short distraction.

For many of us, emotional eating starts young. The reason it happens is that one day you find yourself in a situation where you feel very strong emotions, but there is nothing you can do, no action you can take, to resolve them. You are truly out of control. It can be a child who is crushed by his parent's divorce, who desperately wants them to stay together, but there is nothing he can do to make that happen or a child forced to move, leaving all his or her friends behind, who is left feeling lost and lonely. It can happen in those times in life when you feel all alone without the support system you need to be able to vent your feelings in a safe, kind place.

Over and over with my worst cases of emotional eating, I hear the word "trapped" over and over again. For example, one woman ended up nearly 300 pounds while she was engaged to an abusive man because she felt she couldn't safely leave. She felt trapped, she turned to food and had the added benefit of ending up so heavy her problem resolved itself. Once her fiancé was gone, the weight started disappearing too.

I've seen it in a mother who lost her son. There was nothing she could do to bring him back and she ate to give herself a moment of peace when she thought of nothing but the food. I've seen it in a woman who felt "trapped" in her job. It was a terrible environment where she dreaded going into work and felt her boss was out to get her. She had a very narrow skill set and couldn't find another job that would pay anywhere near what she was making. She had bills that had to be paid and could see no way to get away from her situation so she consoled herself with mindless eating.

Still, by far, the most common situation for emotional eating is feeling "trapped" in a bad romantic situation. I call it the, "But I Love Him Syndrome." I've heard it all. "I think my husband is bipolar, I never know who I'm going to get when I walk in the door, Dr. Jekyll or Mr. Hyde." "My husband screams at me all the time, he's really nasty and says some horrible things." "My marriage has gone cold. My husband barely looks at me, let alone talks to me. I feel like I'm on my own, feeling isolated and judged in my own home." These women and men are unhappy, miserable even, but feel they don't want to or can't leave. Sometimes it's because kids are involved, sometimes it's about money and sometimes they just aren't ready to let the relationship go.

In all these cases, if there is a terrible situation at the root of their eating, until they take action to resolve the problem, any weight they lose will quickly be regained. Some clients make the necessary changes and lose the weight while others uncover the problem and choose to continue to do nothing about it.

My worst failure as a hypnotist was the woman trapped in her job. She hated it. It was causing her to become fat and miserable but, because she'd applied for other jobs and had found nothing, she refused to take any further action. She spent large amounts of money to hire a personal trainer for two days a week, hired me for six sessions of hypnosis, got a personalized dietitian-designed eating program from me, then decided to try gluten free, signed up for hot yoga and then joined a professionally run support group for emotional eaters. She spent thousands of dollars on different things, paid her money and showed up. I explained for her that the scale does not care about good attendance. She never lost more than a few pounds without the weight coming back.

We ended with me explaining her situation to her and pointing out there are always options; yet she still refused to do anything to address the root of her emotional eating. Emotional eaters are the toughest nuts to crack, the toughest cases to turn around. They routinely come in weighing the most of any of my clients. I have noticed that almost all the individuals who come in my door weighing 240 pounds or more are emotional eaters.

As I explained to one client, most people don't down half a large pan of cinnamon rolls and an entire half gallon of milk. When that's going on, it's not about cravings, it's not about an incorrect sense of portion size or what your body needs, it's about emotions being pushed down with food.

That's not to say that I haven't seen tons of emotional eaters, lose tons of weight and rediscover their emotions and take action address those emotions. One woman realized her husband had a psychological problem and resolved to get him the medical help he needed. Another woman had a boss she didn't get along with; she walked into her boss's office one day and had a heart to heart talk about what was wrong and how the situation could get better. Was it perfect? No, but it was acknowledged and addressed. And, by the way, that woman was down 40 pounds the last time I heard from her.

Another woman dealing with emotional eating issues had aborted three babies when she was young; she felt horrible guilt and sadness. She eventually went on retreat for women who were grieving over their decisions to have abortions in the past. She realized she wasn't alone, even had a memorial service for the children she had decided not to have and, most importantly, found forgiveness for herself. Weight that hadn't budged for decades started coming off.

You see, when it comes to emotional eating, the pattern is

feel an emotion and eat…feel an emotion and eat… feel an emotion and eat. I believe the best metaphor for this I've ever found was in one of my favorite books on Eriksonian hypnosis. It points out that emotional eating is like driving a car. You see the oil light go on and then you put more gas in the car. Then noticing the oil light is still on, pulling into another gas station and adding a gas can in your back seat. This happens over and over again and soon your back seat is full of gas cans, your trunk is full of gas cans and your oil light is still on. It's not until the car starts really having problems that it finally ends up at the mechanics. For some people the mechanic is a heart bypass or treatment for diabetes, for others it's consulting me or someone like me. To help someone get past emotional eating you have to help them realize their emotions are just like that oil light or any other warning light on their car. They're not meant to be ignored. They are an early warning system that needs to be noticed and addressed directly, only then will the oil light turn off.

Emotions are like your sixth sense. They clue you in that you need something or that something is wrong. If you're lonely you need to recognize it and find someone to talk to. If you're angry, you need to admit it to yourself and find some way to get that anger released. Sometimes it's appropriate to share it with the person causing the anger, at other times you just need to vent to someone else or write about your feelings in a journal. Sometimes dealing with emotions takes a very, very vigorous house cleaning or a strong, brisk walk around the block. Sadness needs to be recognized and addressed as well and discussed with someone who can give emotional support. If it's an ongoing situation, action may need to be taken to create some relief, if possible. You have to do the emotional work, if you are an emotional eater. There is no way around it.

The problem isn't that you haven't found the "right" diet yet. The problem isn't that you can't find the time to go to the gym or just haven't discovered a work out you enjoy. The diet doesn't matter. Adkins, Gluten-Free, The Zone, South Beach or dietitian created. They will all work! Yes, some are better than others, but as long as your calories out are greater than the calories you're taking in, you will lose weight. The problem is not finding the "right" diet or "your" form of exercise.

The problem is that emotions in your life are causing you to be out of control and eat large amounts of food. Those large amounts of food contain large amounts of calories which cause you to gain weight and undo any weight loss progress you've made. It's not about how perfect you can be on the best diet on the planet. It's about all those times when the food is being shoveled into your mouth, without you noticing how much you're eating or even what it tastes like. That's what is causing you to be overweight. That's what is keeping the weight on. That's what has to change for you to lose the weight and keep it off forever!

PUT YOURSELF ON THE MENU

I'm just going to say it. People, it's time to stop being your own last priority! Whether it is work, family, friends, hobbies or just household chores, so many people make themselves and their health come in last. They get too little sleep and have too much stress and instead of giving their bodies what they really need, like a rest, they just continue to try to fuel up with extra calories.

They "reward" themselves with sugar and quick burning carbs trying to find the energy and the will to force themselves through the day. Just STOP! Instead of giving themselves a break from the kids, a vacation from work, a way to unwind, people are giving themselves a reward during the day, or at the end of a long day, that comes in the form of a fast or sweet treat—think French fries, soda pop, cookies, candy, etc. Sound familiar? Often they don't even sit down long enough to really savor it.

Too much stress, too little sleep and too little caring about your own health can derail any attempt at weight loss before it even starts. Too little sleep makes you tired, more in need of quick energy, with a subconscious that is running the show because your conscious mind is basically asleep. If your subconscious is programmed to eat junk, that is exactly what you'll do. Too much stress makes it nearly impossible to eat well, even though that's what you need the most to help get through a tough situation. Instead, people often turn to sweets or junk food as a reward or as a coping mechanism. For long-term weight loss to be successful, you must first address sleep and stress issues and fix them as much as possible because they will destroy your weight loss efforts before they even begin.

ARE YOU GENEROUS OR STINGY WITH YOURSELF?

One way to discover exactly how generous or stingy you are being with yourself and your health is to do an activity called the weight loss bank. It forces you to assign a monetary number to your weight loss goal and then pay yourself for each daily step you take to achieve that goal.

If you aren't paying yourself very much, it becomes obvious that you aren't being generous with your own needs and making your health a priority. Here is how it works: The Weight Loss Bank has proven successful in helping thousands of people make real changes in their life. It works on a subconscious level and takes advantage of special features of the human mind to bypass your conscious mental filter, to help you reprogram your subconscious.

The Weight Loss Bank idea was inspired by The Mental Bank concept that was created by Dr. John Kappas. He was a widely respected psychologist and one of the founders of modern hypnotherapy. After many decades of work as a hypnotherapist, he was looking for a way people could most successfully make changes to their own subconscious. He tried subliminal tapes and straightforward positive thinking. He was experimenting on his clients and found both methods gave them little success. Then, using his understanding of the special features of the human brain, he developed the Mental Bank which takes advantage of handwriting and precognitive dreams to effectively reprogram the brain. He then studied the results of its long term use on thousands of people and found those who did it religiously achieved incredibly positive results toward reaching their goals.

The first step in creating your own Weight Loss Mental Bank is to find your goal weight and decide exactly how many pounds you want to lose. You then write down, using your own handwriting (not the computer), your weight loss goals. For example your goal, if you are a medium sized woman, your goal might be 130 pounds. If you currently weigh 180 pounds that means you need to lose 50 pounds. So each night you would write your goal as 130 pounds with a weight loss of 50 pounds.

This first step is one of the most important. Just by writing those two numbers you are familiarizing yourself with seeing 130 pounds and with that being your correct weight. You see, one of the major difficulties people have in weight loss is self sabotage. It slows their weight loss progress and leads to them regain the weight they have lost. Remember, to your subconscious the unknown is a painful thing. Your mind wants to stay comfortable right where you are. It is an idea known as homeostasis. It is the reason we stay at a job we hate much longer than we should because we are afraid of what will happen if we try to make a change. It is also the reason we may ignore certain medical symptoms, skipping a much-needed doctor's visit because we are afraid of what the doctor might find. It is our fear of the unknown that is holding us back every time. It also can lead us to unconscionably hold on to weight because we subconsciously see weighing less as frightening.

The next step is to turn your weight loss goal into a financial number, so you can easily see the progress you are making towards your goal and get credit for the work you are doing. Long term weight loss isn't about numbers on a scale, which can be impacted by water weight and muscle creation. Long term weight loss is about making long term lifestyle changes, by living those changes every day and making them part of your daily habits. It is about changing the way you think, so you automatically live better and keeping those life changes becomes easier.

The way you monetize your goal weight loss is by simply adding three zeros to the back end of the amount you want to lose. For example, if you want to lose 50 pounds, your goal becomes $50,000. The reason we use financial numbers when doing our Weight Loss Bank work is not only because the human subconscious seems to understand numbers well. Our subconscious is particularly familiar with financial numbers; we deal with money every day with every item we purchase.

By converting your weight loss goal into a financial goal and then logging how much you are earning, you are paying yourself to do the right things to reach your goal. It's an easy way to see how generous or cheap you are being with yourself. Being cheap with yourself is one major characteristic of many people who struggle to maintain healthy habits. While it may seem like they're being overly generous with themselves when it comes to food, often the opposite is true. People tend to overeat to give themselves "treat" food, in place of giving themselves the good nutrition they really need.

For example, say a man is trapped in a job he hates. It leaves him too mentally exhausted and drained to exercise and he is so stressed he turns to junk food. What he really needs is to leave the bad job. He is not generous enough with himself to do what he really needs and get away from the job, no matter the cost. Instead, he is "faux-generous" to himself with food. Another example would be the mother of young children. She is too exhausted to work out at the end of the day after watching the kids all day and too "busy" to pay attention to what she eats. She knows she really needs some time each day just for herself, her health and her goals, but she feels too guilty about leaving her kids, even for a short time. Instead, she is "faux generous" to herself with treats and taking a break from exercise.

When done correctly, the Weight Loss Bank holds people accountable for being cheap with themselves. You just have to make sure you are only paying yourself for the actions that move you towards your goal. For example, write down all the new, healthier choices you made during the day, paying yourself $100 for each of them. Keep this type of log daily for a few months. It will help you notice if you are generous or cheap with yourself and, best of all, by the time you've earned $50,000 you should be close to having lost 50 pounds.

SKINNY SECRET 15: YOU CAN BEAT SELF-SABOTAGE

The final emotional issue that can keep weight on like it was locked to your body is your "secret benefit". Secret benefits are also often referred to as secondary gain. That means, "What exactly are the emotional benefits of keeping the weight on?"

Many women, and even some men, use their weight as a type of shield. It keeps them from getting too much attention. Some feel it helps them blend into the background a bit. This factor is especially true for someone who has been a victim of sexual assault or felt endangered during a romantic relationship. Being overweight is also a great excuse for failure. If you are heavy and someone rejects you and turns you down for a date, you can blame the fat.

Weight can also be an excuse for avoiding going after what you really want in life. In that case, the person says to themselves, "Well, I really need to lose weight before I can go after that dream." Someone who is heavy may also worry about how their personal relationships with friends or romantic partners would change if they began to lose weight. If their spouse is also heavy or likes them to be a bit heavy, the thought of being thinner could be very frightening, especially on an unconscious level.

HYPNOSIS TO BEAT EMOTIONAL EATING

To achieve permanent weight loss, the various types of emotional hang-ups must be dealt with. Using either self or professional hypnosis is a great tool for that.

For example, someone who is using weight as an excuse for avoiding life and going after what they really want must imagine a time in their life when they felt the most confident and strong. They must feel those feelings again and again bringing them forward into their present reality. They can anchor those feeling to an object or part of their body by imaging those feeling going into that object or body part. They can then touch that item to get in touch with those feelings throughout the day. This is known as the "Confidence Technique." Once the person is feeling stronger and more confident, they can begin to go after those dreams before losing all the weight. With their excuses gone, actually losing the weight and keeping it off is likely to be more achievable.

Some people are afraid that losing weight might cause them to lose in their emotional relationships. They, too, can use hypnosis to address their problem. The most successful self-hypnosis to repeat over and over again is known as the Happy Ending technique. Simply imagine successfully losing weight and creating various happy ending scenarios that address whatever specific fear they have about the results of their weight loss. For example, they must imagine or visualize their partner being thrilled for them, impressed by their determination and eventually inspired to create a healthier lifestyle for themselves. One interesting note, what you imagine has often proven to become your actual reality.

Finally, for someone using weight as a shield, those with very real fears from traumatic life experiences, such as sexual assault or issues of abandonment need more in-depth therapy with a psychologist who has plenty of experience treating their type of trauma. For others who use weight as a shield in order to blend in, the "Confidence Technique" can be used very effectively. The technique will create a new beneficial shield to help "protect" them from the world. In hypnosis, they need to imagine or visualize an invisible shield surrounding them helping to protect them. They can also bring themselves back to a time when they felt most safe and comfortable in their own body and then work to anchor those feeling to an object or part of their body by imaging those feeling going into that object or body part. They can then touch that item to get in touch with those feelings throughout the day.

FINISHING UP: FIND YOUR TIPPING POINT

Guess what? You don't have to follow all of the exercises and suggestions mentioned in this book to lose weight. It's OK if you only want to do 8, or only 2, of the 15 Mental Secrets. You just need to make enough of an effort to hit your tipping point. What's a tipping point? It's Malcolm Gladwell's idea that there is a "tipping point" to every major change. A point at which trend, product or new way of thinking suddenly catches on and then spreads with a life of its own.

This is the recipe for how lasting change works. It involves a process, which may happen over a number of months or even years. Here's how it works… you get new information, your circumstances change, you do your emotional homework to grow, you have external factors or other people helping guide you. Then, there comes that second when it all comes together. That moment when enough has finally happened to create a major, lasting change in your life.

That is why someone who as "failed" time and again at losing weight and keeping it off can, at some point, succeeds long term. What I'm describing is like an actor who has honed his craft for years, who then suddenly gets a break out role that makes him an "overnight success." My point is that YOU can have that break out moment, too. What can seem like almost magical long-term weight loss is really just an accumulation of small shifts in someone's behavior and thought process that suddenly reaches a tipping point. Then it tips that person into thinking and behaving like a thin person, which makes and keeps them thin.

Suddenly, they find themselves with more control over their trigger foods, eating smaller portions, moving more, suffering from bad emotional eating choices less often, and having more healthy foods readily available. My point is this; the secret to their success wasn't getting a personal trainer, finding the "right" diet for them, discovering a magic little pill or getting hypnotized one time by some onstage magician. Instead, the magic was in those small shifts; a habit change, weight loss hypnosis, cutting calories, a shift in thinking... that each happened one baby step at a time. Those baby steps are totally sustainable and can last a lifetime.

HOW I KNOW IT WORKS

This "Tipping Point" truth makes me think of my most successful clients. They often come in after trying every fad diet, every crazy hormone or pill, every weight loss program and latest workout trend. Nothing has worked for them. The "crazy" idea of trying hypnosis is their absolute last resort. They are rather skeptical. Some hope one session will work like magic. I try to explain what's going on with them. Why they keep failing over and over again, no matter what they try. The problem is that they are thinking, acting and living like overweight people who desperately want to be thin. They go from trend to trend, fad to fad... with a lot of bad eating, couch sitting and feeling bad about their weight. To successfully lose weight and keep it off, the secret is all in the amount of effort you put in. Living like a thin person, eating like a thin person and thinking like a thin person will, over time, cause you to become a thin person.

This is the best, most complete advice I can offer based on what I have learned over my entire career in fitness, weight loss and hypnosis. Please, make a few of the small changes I recommend to your personal environment and you will naturally eat better and eat less. Cut down on sugar and you will cut down on your cravings for junk food. Buy my weight loss hypnotherapy recordings or simply try my self hypnosis methods spelled out in this book. If done correctly, you will likely begin to notice more control over your cravings and eating habits. Explore the emotional reasons behind bad eating choices by noticing how you are feeling and what you are doing when those bad choices are made. Each small step will bring you closer and closer to being in lasting control of your weight.

You can do this! I've helped hundreds of people find lasting weight loss and I've passed my best techniques along to you. Now is the time to put some effort into yourself and your health. You have the tools and the information. Now it's up to you!

ADDENDUM: SECRETS TO SELF HYPNOSIS

To reprogram someone's mind, or your own mind, just strip away the critical thinking function of the conscious mind. Movies do this by getting you caught up in a great story, your imagination does this by getting you caught up in a detailed fantasy, and your car does this on long road trips by overloading your senses with lots of fast moving stimuli until you mentally just shut down letting your unconscious take over. Hopefully, you're a good driver.

In the opposite case, if you just walked up to heavy people on the street and told them that the second you snapped your fingers they would suddenly love exercise and hate junk food it wouldn't work. The actor with the chainsaw works in the movies and the image of horrible accident works when you're worrying because it's bypassing your critical thinking. Since the person on the street is not in hypnosis, the idea of loving exercise and hating sweets would be rejected because their critical thinking functions are fully intact. It would reject those ideas as a lie. They would tell themselves that they really hate sweating it out at the gym and would polish off a box of cookies entirely on their own if given the chance.

Hypnosis works because, like long road trips, movies and day dreams, it dials down your critical thinking abilities so ideas can actually penetrate into your subconscious. It uses deep relaxation to put people in a daydream like state, similar to the feeling you have right before falling asleep and just as you are waking up. That is the state in which people experience vivid imaginary events that seem to be very real to them. Their conscious mind turns off, ignoring the reality around them and allows them to escape into another place. Their mind accepts these images as real and then their body experiences them as if they were really happening. Their heart rate speeds up; chemicals are released in their brain, just the same as if a dramatic event were actually taking place at that moment.

However, just like when watching a movie or daydreaming,

when in hypnosis you are really in control the entire time. It is impossible to enter hypnosis unwillingly. To be hypnotized a person has to make a decision that they want to relax and allow their mind to drift off. To exit hypnosis a person can generally get themselves wide awake just by focusing on becoming more alert, then counting to 10 and opening their eyes.

HOW TO DO SELF HYPNOSIS

If you are going to attempt to harness the power of hypnosis, you should also know self-hypnosis or using a hypnotherapy recording often works best right before bed. This is a time many people do not feel as rushed and are used to relaxing their bodies to achieve a state similar to hypnosis right before they drift off to sleep. Most hypnotherapy recordings will have an induction into hypnosis built in, so all you have to do is just press play.

Sometimes, however, when you have less time, want to deal with a specific personal issue, or want to get into a deeper state of trance, it is better to use self-hypnosis. To hypnotize themselves, a person can either let their mind begin to wander and, as they get close to sleep, direct their thoughts to new beliefs, images or changes they want to have in their lives. Even better, they might consciously do a self-hypnosis and direct their thoughts, once they are in a light hypnosis, until they fall asleep. To get yourself into a state of hypnosis, stare at one small spot on the wall or a small light on an appliance. This is called an eye fascination. You will eventually feel a desire to close your eyes, when you do feel that desire, please close them. Then, while lying down, perform what is called a progressive body relaxation. Start with your feet feeling very heavy and relaxed and move all the way through your body and up to your head. Let that warm, heavy feeling move through your entire body, relaxing every muscle it touches.

You could also imagine a warm healing light or a golden healing liquid pouring into your body, relaxing every muscle. Notice how your body is feeling relaxed, floaty, tingly... pick a describing word and you can use it next time you do self-hypnosis to become more deeply hypnotized even more quickly. Count backward for yourself now from 10 down to 0, feeling more and more relaxed as the numbers descend. Notice your breathing getting deeper, slower and more rhythmic. Now picture yourself walking down a stairway or a beautiful sloping path. Imagine all the details you see around you as you descend down the staircase or path. There are 20 steps on the staircase, imagine getting healthier or closer to your ideal body image with each step you take.

Remember, everyone has experienced hypnosis before in one form or another. It is that feeling of losing track of time and external pressures that you hope to achieve during hypnosis. The more you practice it, the better you will become at entering hypnosis and the more effective it will become.

Please remember though, never use a hypnotic recording or attempt to go into self-hypnosis while driving or doing anything else where your complete attention is required. If you ever find yourself in a hypnotic state while doing any of these activities please count yourself out of hypnosis. You count up from 0 to 10, becoming more wide awake as the numbers go up. It is also helpful for some people if they snap their fingers near their ear once they reach 10. This is a great way to quickly return to a wide awake state and signal your conscious mind that it is time to become fully alert.

THE ROLE OF SELF HYPNOSIS

Self-hypnosis can be very helpful for people with the determination to practice it repeatedly. If done correctly, it can allow you to gain access to your subconscious and make long-term behavior changes. Self-hypnosis is so effective many hypnotherapists use it as part of each session. They take a few moments to give clients a chance to reflect on suggestions and find how those suggestions best relate to them personally.

They also have clients practice self-hypnosis at home, along with using professional guided hypnosis recordings. It is a common belief of many hypnotherapists that their clients often know best how to solve their own deepest problems and only need to be guided to find those solutions. This was an idea first introduced by the famous psychologist and hypnotherapist, Milton Erikson. He is widely recognized as one of the founders of modern psychology.

There are two issues though that makes pure self-hypnosis difficult to achieving maximum effectiveness. It takes a great deal of practice do well and is never the same as professional hypnosis. You see, when going into a hypnotherapist's office, the therapist will try to overload your mind with information and questions to cause your mind to escape into hypnosis. This is a process of disorganizing your thoughts so, once they get you into a very relaxed state, a hypnotherapist has access to put in their own suggestions. Then, they do the reprogramming for you by telling you what to think, visualize or imagine. For many, this allows professionals to get them more deeply into hypnosis and get them results more quickly.

The exact reverse of this process is true for self-hypnosis. A person in self-hypnosis has to organize their own thoughts and continue using part of their conscious mind to guide their thoughts to create the right mental experiences to help themselves make permanent changes. Still, self-hypnosis can be very effective, as proven by brain scans showing people's bodies experiencing their daydreams as reality. In order for it be most effective, a person has to really be in touch with what ideas they need to reprogram and then have a plan for how to successfully create better ideas while in self-hypnosis.

Sometimes a person can realize better than anyone else what images or messages they need to make a permanent life-style change. Often though, hypnosis isn't a one shot deal and using weight loss hypnotherapy recordings or going to a professional hypnotherapist's office is helpful.

ABOUT THE AUTHORS

Allison and Ryan Staley are the creators and owners of Fitnotism in
Las Vegas, NV. They also own three Snap Fitness Franchise
locations. They have nearly 3 decades of experience in the fitness
and weight loss industry.
Both are certified personal trainers and certified master hypnotists.
They have graduated from the Hypnosis Motivation Institute, which
is the only nationally accredited school for hypnosis is the country.
They have used hypnosis to help hundreds of clients lose weight and
regain their health.